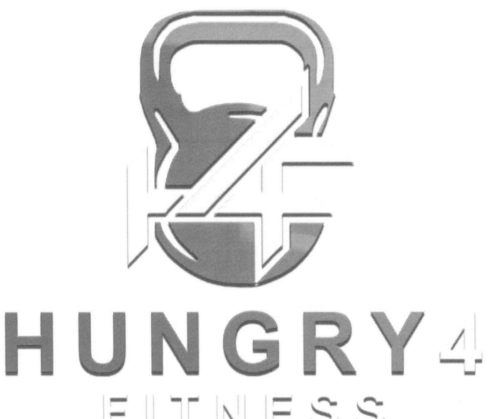

HUNGRY4
FITNESS

FIRST EDITION

Health Disclaimer

In memory of
Lee

Contents

Introduction
What's new in Volume 2?
Essential training principles

Workouts 1 to 10
1. Six Sizzling AMRAPs
2. Kettlebell HIIT
3. 20-Minute Body Weight Bonanza
4. 30-Minute Cardio & Calisthenics Corker
5. Spartan *300* Workout
6. Kettlebell & Cardio
7. Dumbbell HIIT
8. Hill Sprints
9. One Barbell & Four Compound Exercises
10. Fat-loss Circuit

Workouts 11 to 20
11. 300 Kettlebell Swings
12. 500 Kettlebell Swings
13. 1300 Repetitions
14. 10 X 2-Minute AMRAPs
15. Cardio & Calisthenics Scorcher
16. The Perfect Way to Start the Day
17. The Ultimate Sandbag Session
18. Dumbbell Leg *Explosion!*
19. 30-Minute Barbell Complex
20. From Russia with Love

Workouts 21 to 30
21. Buy One Get Two Free
22. Military Combat Training
23. 21 CrossFit WODs
24. Compound Exercise Pyramid
25. Strength & Fitness Conditioning
26. Smash it for 7-Minutes
27. 20-Minute Kettlebell Circuit
28. Kettlebell & Body Weight Pyramids
29. *Go Hercules!*
30. High-Intensity Interval Training

Workouts 31 to 40
31. Classic Kettlebell Competitions
32. Three Measly Minutes
33. 10-Minute HIIT
34. A Compendium of CrossFit EMOMs
35. The Kettlebell Snatch
36. Skip and Swing Sesh
37. EMOM Madness
38. Boxing Cardio & Calisthenics Combo
39. High-Intensity Interval Skipping
40. 4-Week Strongman Training Programme

Workouts 41 to 50
41. The Power of Fitness Testing
42. 10,000 Kettlebell Swing Challenge
43. Train Like a Martial Arts Legend

44. Boxing Met-Con Mania

45. 10-Ton Upper Body Strength
Challenge

46. 10-Ton Lower Body Strength
Challenge

47. Functional Fitness Training

48. Train Hard Fight Easy!

49. Five More EMOMs

50. The Grand Finale: Marathon Row

Appendix A – Circuit and Workout
Design
Appendix B – Stretching Plan
References

'Circuit training is . . . a way of developing all-round fitness. Decreases in body fat and increases in strength, as assessed by the one repetition maximum effort, and maximum oxygen uptake have been reported as a result of circuit training.'

– A. W. S. Watson
Physical Fitness & Athletic Performance

Why start circuit training?

Circuit training is one of the best forms of physical exercise for maintaining and increasing overall fitness. A well-designed circuit will provide a great cardiovascular workout, strengthening the heart and lungs in the process, while also improving muscle endurance and building functional strength.

This dual fat-burning and muscle-building combination, which single exercises – such as running, cycling, swimming, or weightlifting – cannot confer, will help to sculpt a lean defined physique.

The versatility of circuits is such that they can be constructed so as to place emphasis on a specific component of fitness – strength, muscular endurance, coordination, agility – or to enhance sport performance. For example, if you enjoyed boxing and wanted to improve your pugilism as well as your fitness, you could tailor a circuit to incorporate boxing-specific movements or include the punch bag as a station. (See Workouts 38 and 44 for examples.)

Circuits can be conducted in solitary or social settings. Because of the inherent flexibility of circuits, they can be adapted to accommodate multiple trainers of varying physical abilities. In a well-designed circuit, you could have an advanced trainer exercising alongside a complete beginner and they would both still be able to maximise their respective abilities – neither impeding the other.

Solitary circuits are a great way to get a lot done in a short space of time. You can throw together a mixture of exercises – best to do this with as little thought as possible – and for 20-plus-minutes try to complete as many repetitions and cover as many metres as your physicality will permit. High-intensity circuit training such as I've crudely outlined will 'overload the cardiovascular system and result in an increase in aerobic capacity,' (Watson 1995).

Benefits of circuit training

- They can be tailored to a specific sport, increasing the individual's fitness, and sharpening their skill set at the same time.
- Circuits can provide a means of testing fitness or be used for competition among multiple trainers.
- They are bewilderingly versatile; the number of layouts and exercises that can be included should ensure that the trainer has a new and different workout every week for life.
- Circuits allow the trainer to shoehorn a lot of exercise into a short space of time. This attribute makes them perfect for the person with a predilection for productivity.
- They enable the trainer to target multiple components of fitness simultaneously in the same workout. Circuits can be constructed to 'emphasise different aspects of fitness such as strength, muscular endurance, speed, [and even] flexibility' (Watson, 1995).
- And finally, as already stated, circuits are an excellent exercise modality for burning fat and sculpting a lean, defined physique.

So, what is a circuit?

Distilled down to its essence, a circuit could be defined simply as a physical training session that incorporates multiple exercises where the trainer performs as many repetitions or loops as possible in a pre-specified period.

The classical conception of the circuit is that of a loop or circle of exercises that an individual or group carries out in rotation. However, this is an outdated and quite parochial perception of what constitutes a circuit. They can take on a multitude of different forms and the exercises from which the circuit is comprised do not have to be merely calisthenics and/or light resistance.

The combination and types of exercises that can be included within a circuit are limited only by the imagination of the trainer. In some of the circuits throughout the **Hungry4Fitness** *Book of Circuits Vol. 2*, you will see an arbitrary assortment of exercises that present the appearance of having been cobbled together extemporaneously. And while this is in part the case, when it comes to circuit design, I've found that being rigorously prescriptive often results in a dull, monotonously mechanistic exercise experience. Truly, spontaneity in selecting exercises can spice up a workout making it both refreshing and physically rewarding.

Concerning conventionality of correct training, as far as I am aware there is no universal law prohibiting a strength exercise following hot on the heels of, say, a cardiovascular blast on the running machine, or a row sprint into a series of kettlebell snatches. If anything, a circuit designed in this way is more reflective of most all competitive sports and realistic of the demands of life.

So, when designing a circuit, really you ought to shrug off the constrictive straitjacket of convention. It is perfectly acceptable – nay! *preferable* – to mix 'conflicting' components of fitness or pair together exercises that stimulate the same muscle groups. Truly, circuit training is the ultimate no-holds-barred exercise arena where anything goes.

What you can get from this book

It may not have escaped your notice, but most people who go to the gym, who participate in some form of physical exercise or another, do not achieve much. From one year to the next most trainers make no physical improvements, and their physiques remain the same. Why is that? Why is it that even consistently committed exercisers fail to experience the fruits of their physical labours?

One prevailing misconception that I continue to encounter is that participating in physical exercise is enough. You yourself may have heard it said that to lose weight and get fit all you've got to do is *go to the gym*. It matters not what you do or the intensities at which you train, going is enough. As though gyms are imbued with some magical fat-loss, fitness-promoting power that is instantly bestowed on those who pass through the doors.

Of course, this is pure poppycock. Going to the gym, even actually *exercising* at the gym, does not guarantee aesthetical and physical improvement. This salient fact has slipped beneath the radar of innumerable disgruntled fitness enthusiasts who failed to obtain their idealised selves. *Why*, many a gym-goer has asked themselves in a state of exasperation, *why after all these years of exercising am I still overweight and unfit?*

Truth is, to chisel out a sculpted form from the recalcitrant biological rock, requires years of dedication and persistent hard work. There are few shortcuts to achieving this end and those that are available are arguably undesirable. The same can be said of improving physical fitness: increasing your maximal lift by but a couple of kilograms, say, or shaving off a few seconds from your 10k run time, takes a ton of sweat, tears and toil – and yes, even a few droplets of blood must be spilled from time to time.

To bring this discussion back to the opening gambit, one reason that accounts for why many gym-goers and committed fitness enthusiasts do not improve is that they rarely if ever step outside their training comfort zone. In addition, the majority of exercisers stick to the same old routines: on walking into the gym, they mentally switch off as their autopilot switches on. Physical development and positive changes in body composition will not just come by proxy of participation. They must be *worked* for.

The sad sorry state delineated above is largely a consequence of the failure to produce a pre-workout training plan and the absence of the pursual of fitness goals. In plain English, a plan improves exercise productivity while a goal gives us something to strive for – both powerful motivational forces.

The plethora of circuits and workouts that comprise this book will provide a goal, an objective, and a direction. The difference that can be made to a person's training intensity, because they have a piece of paper with a session plan written on it, is remarkable. Having something to aim for sends enthusiasm and determination levels through the roof. A pre-planned training session can turn an unproductive gym session into a highly productive and rewarding experience.

Who can benefit from this book?

1. **Fitness enthusiasts of all levels who desire a challenge** – due to their innovative designs and cross-training nature, the circuits are more than adequate to provide a challenge for all levels of fitness.
2. **Trainers who have lost motivation and inspiration** – loss of motivation is usually caused by a lack of direction. The absence of a training goal can result in stagnation and a decline in participation. Here, within this book, you will find your lost motivation. I am positive that the circuits and workouts to follow will provide you with a source of inspiration and aid you in discovering a new direction on your physical fitness journey.
3. **Individuals preparing for Armed Forces recruitment** – if you are currently training for the rigours of Armed Forces selection, you will undoubtedly know that superior fitness is of paramount importance. Unlike the recruitment process for civilian jobs, all prospective military recruits must undertake and pass a barrage of fitness tests. The circuits and workouts presented in this book are perfectly suited for forging the fitness needed to meet those physical challenges. In addition, Workout 41 invites you to pit yourself against multiple fitness tests, some of which you will meet throughout military recruitment.
4. **People who want to develop whole-body fitness** – as we discussed in the opening paragraph, circuit training incorporates a broad range of fitness

components. Consequently, it is one of the most effective training methodologies for cultivating complete physicality. Including at least two circuits in your weekly exercise routine will help improve strength, muscle endurance and cardiovascular performance.

5. **Boxers, martial artists, and MMA practitioners** – individuals who practice and/or compete in the combative arts need an abundance of strength, muscular endurance, and cardiovascular fitness. If a mixed martial artist, for example, is lacking in one of these areas they are sure to be exposed at some point during their fight career. Using these circuits and workouts as pre-fight/competition training will help you get in top shape before a contest. Thus, even if you're forced to go the distance, you'll have the fitness to do so.

What's new in Volume 2?

First, Volume 2 contains significantly more circuits and workouts than its predecessor. Yes, there are 50 titles listed on the contents page. However, a good many of those individual titles feature multiple circuits and workouts. For example, number 34, A Compendium of CrossFit EMOMs, has four separate workouts for you to try. And under number 47, you'll discover a whole week's worth of functional fitness training. In short, there is enough exercise entertainment here to keep even the most fanatical of fitness fanatics occupied.

In addition to the veritable wealth of workouts in this book, a number of contemporary training methodologies feature throughout the following pages. As well as an army of AMRAPs and a mob of EMOMs, you'll find CrossFit-inspired barbell complexes, Girevoy kettlebell challenges, boxing conditioning circuits, and even an adaptation of Bruce Lee's 'Total Fitness Routine'. Truly, this book of circuits and workouts must be one of the most comprehensive training tools yet produced.

But the scope of Volume 2 encompasses so much more than just workouts. While the practical application of exercise forms the bulk of the book, there is a fine theoretical thread running throughout. Some workouts come accompanied by a brief outline of the various fitness benefits they aim to bestow. Others offer instructive training advice concerning how to maximise personal performance when undertaking a fitness challenge.

So, in answer to the opening question *What's new in Volume 2?* a lot!

Explanation of the circuit/workout layout

In a bid to mitigate confusion, below I have recreated an example of the exact layout of the circuits and workouts. It might be worth familiarising yourself with the layout so that you do not either miss out essential exercises or worse, include more into the main session than you need to. Both eventualities may adversely affect the mechanics of the workout.

Name and number of the workout

Some circuits and workouts open with a brief introduction. The topic of conversation is typically concerned with outlining the fitness benefits the workout bestows. But sometimes the introduction aims to enlighten the reader on the mechanics and training methodologies employed. The purpose here is to lay the foundation of understanding for the circuit and workout explanation – or **How it works**.

Below the introduction, you will find out **How it works.** This provides a concise encapsulation of the circuit and how it should be completed. Included within this section (underneath and labelled **key points**) is a bullet-pointed breakdown of all the key elements within the circuit explanation.

Following the overview, some workouts feature a section that succinctly outlines a range of **methods of modification**. The objective here is to provide a few ideas regarding how the workout can be restructured to suit different levels of fitness and training ability.

Mandatory warm-up. Best training practice necessitates a pre-workout warm-up. Thus, every circuit and workout contained in this book begins with a comprehensive and progressive 10-minute warm-up. Of course, the decision is entirely yours if you decide to skip the warm-up. However, to reduce injury risk and improve exercise performance, it is advisable to complete this essential training principle. It's worth remembering that our 'muscles respond better to exercise if they are properly prepared for the coming workload,' (Bean, 2008). The importance of warming up prior to exercise is explained more fully below.

Workout. This section contains the body of the workout. The exercises that feature throughout the workout will be numbered (sometimes bullet-pointed). Those exercises that are likely to present a technical challenge, such as complex compound movements, or quasi-Olympic lifts, are accompanied by an explanation outlining essential technique points.

Cool-down. Some, not all, of the circuits will include a post-workout cool-down.

General advice. Included within this section you will discover a list containing interesting information concerning such things as participatory rules and how certain exercises are to be performed. In addition, advice will be advanced regarding how best to approach the workout. For example, if it enhances training efficiency to organise the exercises in a certain way, or if physical performance will be aided by using progression trackers, I will endeavour to disclose that information.

Circuit/workout modification

The circuits are geared towards an advanced level. However, this does not mean that they cannot be accessed by beginners or intermediate trainers. All the circuits can be modified or adapted to suit your current fitness level and any exercise that features within a circuit can be substituted for one that is preferable.

The circuits and workouts were completed in a public gym/leisure complex making them more accessible to a wider audience. However, many of them can be adapted to home gyms or to accommodate a dearth of exercise equipment.

Training principles

The following few pages outline the three essential training principles: warm-up, cool-down, and stretching. In addition to touching on the importance of each principle, a summative outline of the approach protocol is provided. Advanced trainers may want to skip this section. However, brushing up on fitness fundamentals is beneficial for beginners and experienced trainers alike.

Warm-up

All the circuits and workouts include a simple 10-minute warm-up. Warm-ups have been included to better prepare you for the training session and to reduce injury susceptibility. Failing to warm-up prior to exercise, even if the workout is low-intensity or involves static weightlifting, increases injury risk factor. As well as reducing injury risk a progressive whole-body warm-up enhances physical performance. It does this by raising the body's core temperature and facilitating neuromuscular function.

Warming up also prepares you psychologically for physical activity. The two most common barriers to exercise that many trainers struggle to surmount include flagging motivation and a general loss of appetite. Sometimes it can be a real effort to get to the gym or go out for that run. However, what we often find (once we've eventually dragged ourselves to the gym or laced up our trainers) is that after a good warm-up we are ready and raring for exercise.

You need only spend 10-minutes warming up prior to a training session. For the warm-ups that precede each circuit and workout, follow the simple process below.

Although the following example has been tailored to suit a running session, the same underlying process can be applied to circuits, cycling, rowing, and any other form of physical training.

10-minute progressive warm-up
- 2-minutes walking and gentle mobility exercises
- Ease into a slow jog
- 3-minutes low-intensity jogging
- Stop and complete 10 repetitions of the following three exercises: squats, burpees, and squat thrusts (30- to 45-seconds)
- Begin jogging again for a further 2-minutes but now increase the intensity – the increase should be progressive and barely perceptible
- Stop and complete 20 repetitions of the same body weight exercises (1-minute)
- Carry on jogging for the remaining time and progressively build the pace to that of the run.

(This warm-up will naturally integrate into the main workout, which is precisely what a good warm-up should do.)

The above process is supposed to provide a simplistic sketch of a progressive warm-up. However, you should always ensure to complete one similar prior to participating in physical exercise. Of course, I am not suggesting that you use the exact exercises above, just the methodology: gradually building up the intensity while ensuring that the exercises within the warm-up closely reflect those that feature in the main session.

Should I stretch during the warm-up?
There are, as with most professional bodies, opposing schools of thought within the exercise community concerning what constitutes correct warm-up protocol. Some argue that stretching should be included within the warm-up while others staunchly maintain that it shouldn't. I'm of the opinion that stretching prior to exercise does not negate potential injury risk but can impede physical performance.

In her book *Strength Training | A Complete Guide To*, Anita Bean brings our attention to research that suggests that 'stretching before you start training is unlikely to benefit your performance and, ironically, may even reduce your strength and increase the risk of injury.' This shouldn't come as a surprise when we remember that stretching, more accurately *static stretching*, is essentially a restorative relaxation technique. It goes without saying that, before attempting a tough physical challenge, it would be unwise to perform a series of relaxing movements.

Furthermore, by stopping mid-warm-up to stretch, the body will begin to cool thus defeating the primary purpose of warming up. A progressive warm-up, like the example outlined above, that builds in intensity over 10-minutes, will adequately prepare you both physically and mentally for the ensuing exercise session.

Warm-up summary

- Ensure the muscles and physiological systems that are to be targeted in the main session form the primary focus of your warm-up. Of course, a warm-up that does not reflect the main session will fail to rouse the requisite physiological responses. It would be almost useless cycling for 10-minutes when your main session consists of an upper-body weights circuit. To recapitulate: a warm-up should consist of a cardiovascular element and exercises that feature throughout the main session.
- Begin your warm-up at a low intensity and progressively increase it across the desired duration.
- Include a cardiovascular element – such as running, skipping, or rowing – in your warm-up. As their name suggests, cardio exercises are most effective at raising heart rate and core temperature.
- The optimum warm-up duration is 10-minutes.
- As discussed above, stretching is not a necessary component of the warm-up protocol. However, with that said, if you would prefer to include a short stretch in your warm-up, it is advisable to do so early on. Stretching near the conclusion of your warm-up will likely result in the decrease of core body temperature, which contravenes the purpose of the process.

- Remember, it is an act of folly to skip the warm-up and the trainer who neglects this crucial phase of the workout increases their risk of sustaining an injury.

Cool-down

After you have completed an arduous workout, it is perfectly natural to lie on the floor for a while and wallow in a pool of sweat and self-pity. But what the consummate professional always does – after the wallowing bit – is to conduct a cool-down. This oft-neglected phase of a workout is a deregulatory process that decreases the heart rate and core temperature while facilitating the dispersal of metabolic waste.

Important though it indubitably is conducting a cool-down couldn't be simpler. For example, rowing a couple of thousand metres, or retracing your steps, in a relaxed manner, back through part of the main session are both right-out-of-the-text-book cool-downs. Alternatively, you could just complete the warm-up in reverse – high to low intensity.

Cool-down summary

- Begin the cool-down at an intensity that is considerably lower than that of the main session.
- Gradually de-escalate training intensity over 5- to 10-minutes.
- On concluding the cool-down, the exercise intensity – whether it be rowing, cycling, swimming, running, or carrying on with the circuit – should resemble that of walking.
- When you are feeling relaxed and you have somewhat recovered from the main session, this then signifies the time to begin the stretch.

Post-workout stretch

When I said it was an act of folly to neglect warming up before a workout, well, the same can be said for neglecting to complete a post-workout stretch. Sufficient emphasis cannot be placed on the importance of flexibility training. In addition to aiding recovery, augmenting our range of movement (ROM), and with it improving physical performance, stretching has been shown to reduce injury susceptibility. It is for these reasons that you should always make time after exercise for a 5- to 10-minute whole-body stretch.

To make life a little easier for you (read: to ensure you have no excuses to omit this important phase from your training session), a 10-minute stretching plan has been provided (see Appendix B). By implementing the plan post-circuit or workout all your major muscle groups will be treated to a stretch. Feel free to include other stretches or modify the plan to suit your personal preferences.

Workout 1
Six Sizzling AMRAPs

How it works

This session couldn't be simpler. After the warm-up you are to start at the first AMRAP: punches on the heavy bag. Your objective: punch the bag as many times as you can in 10-minutes. Once you've unleashed blind fury for 600 seconds you can treat yourself to a 2-minute rest.

During the rest ensure to make a note of how many punches you achieved. The moment 2-minutes has elapsed progress on to the second AMRAP: powerbag bastods into overhead throws. Same objective as before: try to amass as many reps as possible before you run out of time. Rest. Repeat. Rest. Repeat. Rest. Repeat. Rest. Repeat. Finish!

Methods of modification

There are a million and one ways this session could be modified. Depending on equipment availability, any one of the exercises could be replaced without impacting the dynamics of the session. For example, if you don't have access to a boxing bag, hold a pair of light dumbbells and shadowbox instead.

Also, depending on time constraints and/or current fitness levels, the length of each AMRAP could be reduced to, say, 5-minutes. This would still be a tough cookie of a session even if the AMRAP duration was slashed by half.

Alternatively, you could work through each 10-minute AMRAP with a training partner, taking it in turns 1-minute working/1-minute resting. And, finally, the weights for the resistance exercises can be increased/decreased accordingly.

Key points

- Warm-up! And don't just go through the motions either. A comprehensive, progressive warm-up can reduce injury susceptibility and improve physical performance.
- Begin at the first 10-minute AMRAP: punches on the heavy bag.
- Your objective for this session is to amass as many repetitions, metres, and rotation as possible in 10-minutes.
- You are entitled to a 2-minute rest between each AMRAP.

Warm-up

- 10-minutes skipping at varied intensities.
- Intersperse the skipping with body weight exercises and light kettlebell swings – employ a rep range of between 5 to 10.

Workout

- 10-minute AMRAP: Punches on a heavy bag (1464 punches)
- **2-minute rest**
- 10-minute AMRAP: Powerbag (30kg) bastods into overhead throws* (68 reps)
- **2-minute rest**
- 10-minute AMRAP: Kettlebell swing (40kg) (300 reps)
- **2-minute rest**
- 10-minute AMRAP: Rowing (ergo row) (2712m (1:50/500))
- **2-minute rest**
- 10-minute AMRAP: Farmer's walk (2 x 34kg) (440m)
- **2-minute rest**
- 10-minute AMRAP: Skipping (1268 turns)

Cool-down

- 5/10-minutes low-intensity cardio

Total distance at speed = 2712m
Total KG lifted = 43,840
Total reps = 3100

General advice

- When punching, ensure to fully extend the arms and throw the punch from the chin – none of those pathetic half punches, please!
- *Maintain strict form throughout the powerbag bastods into overhead throws. This is a challenging exercise for two reasons. The first: it works pretty much every muscle in the body. Second: it is technically complicated. On completion of the bastod (which is a burpee followed by a press-up if you didn't know), you are to pop the feet either side of the powerbag and, keeping that back nice and straight, perform a sumo deadlift, followed by a hang-clean, followed by an over-head throw. Told you it was complicated. The exercise should be executed in one smooth movement. Good luck!
- There are a couple of kettlebell swing variations. For this circuit you are only required to get that bell above your belly button.
- For the numerically challenged, counting the skips will be as strenuous as the exercise. I advise, after every 50 or 100 rotations, stopping and tallying each set. That way you're less likely to miscount.
- Prior to embarking on the Farmer's walk, mark out a runway ensuring to measure the distance. When I completed this circuit, I spaced colourful cones 10-metres apart and, like a demented pigeon, paced back and forth for 10-minutes. I kept count of the laps and multiplied the final number by 10-metres.

How it works

Before tackling a HIIT workout it's imperative that you warm-up thoroughly first. Of course, warming up is a principle of training and ought to be observed irrespective of the intensity of the workout. Whether you're about to complete a light gym session or attack a CrossFit AMRAP, you should warm-up.

However, warming up is especially important when training at high intensities for the risk of incurring an injury is greater. It's for this reason that this HIIT kettlebell workout features a progressive 10-minute whole-body warm-up. Once you are sufficiently warmed and (hopefully) raring to go, proceed to work through the three high-intensity intervals below.

You'll notice that for the three exercises each HIIT interval is paired with a rest period. This is standard procedure: HIIT/rest – HIIT/rest. But this HIIT kettlebell workout breaks convention. Instead of resting, you are to engage in an active recovery exercise.

So, after attacking each kettlebell HIIT, you are to complete the accompanying body weight exercise for the same duration. Remember, though, the body weight exercise is performed at a low intensity.

Key points
- Complete the progressive 10-minute warm-up.
- Once warmed, work through the three kettlebell-to-body weight HIITs.
- Use the grids provided to keep track of progress.

Warm-up

- 5-minute row/cross-trainer/skipping (select preferable cardio exercise)
- 10 X 20-second cardio-to-body weight exercise intervals: 20-seconds cardio followed by 20-seconds body weight exercise.

Workout

Kettlebell swing

1. Hold the kettlebell between your legs, palms facing inwards, feet a little over shoulder-width apart.
2. Keeping the back straight pull the kettlebell between your legs and, using your glutes, propel the kettlebell forward until it's level with your shoulders.
3. Ensuring to keep your core engaged throughout the movement, allow the kettlebell to return to the start position and repeat.

Kettlebell swing	20s	20s	20s	20s	20s	20s	20s	20s	20s	20s	20s	20s
Air squat	20s	20s	20s	20s	20s	20s	20s	20s	20s	20s	20s	20s

Kettlebell thruster

1. Standing over the kettlebell, take a reverse grip of the handle. In one clean movement upturn the kettlebell and hold it in front of your chest. In this position the base of the kettlebell should be facing the ceiling.
2. Keeping your back straight squat until your knees are in a 90-degree angle.
3. Power out of the squat ensuring to push the kettlebell high above your head.
4. From the outstretched position lower the kettlebell back to your chest while simultaneously sinking into the next squat.

Kettlebell thruster	20s	20s	20s	20s	20s	20s	20s	20s	20s	20s	20s	20s
Plank	20s	20s	20s	20s	20s	20s	20s	20s	20s	20s	20s	20s

Kettlebell alternate arm clean to press cycle

1. Standing over the kettlebell with a shoulder-width stance (or slightly wider), grasp the handle, swing it back and execute a clean. In this position the kettlebell should be resting in the nook of your arm.
2. Taking a shallow dip at the knee use your quadriceps to get a bit of momentum in the kettlebell. Assist the upward flight of the kettlebell with shoulder and arm strength.
3. From here return the kettlebell back to the original start position but ensure to change hands between the legs so that you can perform the next repetition on the opposite side. Keep the cycle going continuously for 20-seconds.

Kettlebell clean to press cycle	20s	20s	20s	20s	20s	20s	20s	20s	20s	20s	20s	20s
Press ups	20s	20s	20s	20s	20s	20s	20s	20s	20s	20s	20s	20s

General advice

- If you do not yet possess the requisite fitness to perform the body weight exercises after each interval, just take a rest. No shame in that whatsoever.
- Either photocopy the snazzy trackers or, as you progress through the HIIT intervals, make a note of the number of sets completed. This, of course, will remind you of how many interval sets you have completed.
- To improve fluidity throughout the workout, keep your countdown timer and tally sheet close to hand so that you can quickly tick off the set and reset the next 20-second interval. Alternatively, stop being a cheapskate and purchase a proper training timer!
- Following on from the point above, to improve transition efficiency between exercises, ensure to locate all your training tools in one area. This shouldn't pose a problem because all you need is a kettlebell and floor mat for the body weight exercises.

Workout 3
20-Minute Body Weight Bonanza

How it works

This 20-minute EMOM workout is as strait-laced as they get. No funny business and no secret surprises. Promise! Just good honest on the minute every minute. And because it's comprised exclusively of body weight exercises, you can do it almost anywhere.

The only piece of kit needed is a pull-up bar. But, if you're completing this workout at home, or on your hols, and there's no pull-up bar in sight, simply swop pull-ups for something else.

Split into 4 X 5-minute individual blocks, you are to begin at the first EMOM which consists of air squats. From there proceed through the twenty 1-minute sets.

EMOM = *every minute on the minute*

An acronym for every minute on the minute, the EMOM training methodology challenges you to complete a specific number of exercise repetitions in less than 60-seconds. The time remaining allows you to recover before the next minute starts. For a comprehensive discussion on EMOM training, see Appendix A.

Key points

- Progress through the twenty 1-minute EMOM sets.
- Before starting the countdown timer, decide how many reps you are going to complete within each minute.
- Remember, if you were a little too ambitious, and after your reps you are left with insufficient recovery time, reduce to a 50:50 work/rest ratio.

Warm-up

- 5-minute slow jog
- 10 X 50-metre run/sprint intervals: on completion of each sprint perform 5 to 10 reps of each of the four body weight exercises

Workout

EMOM 1: 5 X 1-minute air squats (aim for 30 reps on the minute)

EMOM 1: 5 X 1-minute press-ups (aim for 30/40 reps on the minute)

EMOM 1: 5 X 1-minute burpees (aim for 20 reps on the minute)

EMOM 1: 5 X 1-minute pull-ups (aim for 5/10 reps on the minute)

General advice

- Consider the setup before attempting the workout. Make life easier for yourself by creating a tally sheet. By doing so you can keep track of your progress. In addition, if you make a note of your rep ranges, you can have a go at beating them the next time you complete this workout.
- Ensure to set a repeat countdown timer. This way you won't have to fiddle with your clock between rounds.

Workout 4
30-Minute Cardio & Calisthenics Corker

How it works

Following a similar format as above, this workout is split into six separate 5-minute EMOMs. The aim, of course, is to maintain the rep range for all thirty 1-minute rounds.

But, unlike its predecessors, there is a cardiovascular current running throughout this workout. Between each EMOM set, you'll find a 1000-metre quick-paced run.

The objective here, and this is more for advanced trainers or those who want to push themselves, you must attempt to complete the run in under 4-minutes.

As a reward for your hard work on the run, take however many seconds remain on the clock as rest before the next EMOM set. So, if you complete the run in, say, 3:30, you get 30-seconds rest.

Key points

- Complete all thirty 1-minute EMOM rounds.
- Try to stick as close to the suggested rep ranges as possible.
- If you're feeling fit for it, have a go at the 1000-metre run.

Warm-up

- 10-minute slow-paced jog
- Calisthenics pyramid: complete 1 up to 5 reps for each exercise below

Workout

EMOM 1: 5 x 1-minute plank (hold for 40-seconds)
1000-metre run

EMOM 2: 5 x 1-minute squat thrusts (aim for 40 reps on the minute)
1000-metre run

EMOM 3: 5 x 1-minute press-ups (aim for 30/40 reps on the minute)
1000-metre run

EMOM 4: 5 x 1-minute air squat into plyometric jumps (aim for 25 reps on the minute)
1000-metre run

EMOM 5: 5 x 1-minute pull-ups (aim for 10 reps – if you don't have access to a bar, you're on burpees! 20 reps please)
1000-metre run

EMOM 6: 5 x 1-minute burpees! (aim for 20 reps on the minute)

General advice

- Remember, there's no shame in reducing the reps if you find yourself struggling to get through the round.
- This workout can be completed at the gym or your local park. However, if you opt for the latter venue, ensure that the run distance is accurately measured first. Don't want you skimping on metres!

Workout 5
Spartan *300*

How it works

Popularised by the film *300,* the Spartan 300 Workout is a complete training session. The exercises that comprise the workout engage every muscle in your body. In addition, because it was designed to be completed at a high intensity, it also stimulates your cardiovascular system – as well as testing your mental resolve.

Below there are three versions of the 300 Workout. The first, entitled 'original', is the version that the actors completed in preparation for the film. This is the hardest workout and thus requires an advanced level of fitness to complete.

Lined up beside the original workout are the beginner and intermediate versions. Don't feel discouraged if you have to start with either one of these, for they are still both challenging and provide for an excellent whole-body training session.

Remember, because these workouts feature complex functional exercises and are to be completed at near-maximal intensity, it is important to warm-up thoroughly first.

Key points
- Select the workout commensurate with your current level of fitness and strength.
- After a ruddy good warm-up, prepare yourself mentally for the physical onslaught ahead.
- Start a timer and work through the exercises as quickly as possible.

- On completion of the final rep of the final exercise, stop the clock and document your time for prosperity. A space has been provided at the bottom of each workout for that purpose.

Warm-up

- 2000-metre row – increase intensity every 500-metres.
- Concluding the row complete the following body weight pyramids:
- Press-up: 1 up to 5 reps
- Burpees: 1 up to 5 reps
- Kettlebell swing: 1 up to 5 reps

Beginner Spartan Body Weight Workout	Intermediate Spartan 300 Workout	Original Spartan 300 Warrior Workout
1. Body weight Inverted Rows* – 15 reps 2. Body weight Squats – 25 reps 3. Press-ups – 15 reps 4. Jump Jacks – 50 reps 5. Squat Thrusts – 20 reps 6. Close Grip Press-ups – 10 reps 7. Body weight Inverted Rows – 15 reps	1. Pull-ups – 25 reps 2. Dumbbell Deadlifts (2 x 20kg) – 50 reps 3. Press-ups – 50 reps 4. Body weight Squats – 50 reps 5. V-ups – 50 reps 6. Dumbbell Push Press (2 x 12kg) – 50 reps 7. Pull-ups – 25 reps	1. Pull-ups – 25 reps 2. Barbell Deadlifts (60kg) – 50 reps 3. Press-ups – 50 reps 4. 2-foot Box Jumps – 50 reps 5. Floor Wipers – 50 reps 6. Single-Arm Kettlebell Clean & Press (24kg) – 50 reps 7. Pull-ups – 25 reps
Time:	Time:	Time:

General advice

- If you're desirous of setting a competitive time, it's advisable to situate training equipment in close proximity. The few seconds of toil it'll take to do this will pay you back in the sweet fruit of improved performance.
- *The body weight inverted row is a modification of the pull-up. Typically performed on a Smith machine, set the bar at waist height. Manoeuvre yourself so that you are hanging from the bar with your feet outstretched and planted on the floor. In this position, pull up until your chest touches the bar. Lower back down under control in preparedness for the next repetition.
- The pull-ups must be performed to full extension and no 'kipping'.
- The 50 reps for the single-arm kettlebell clean and press is split 25/25 across both arms. You are permitted to change hands after each completed rep.
- True Spartans complete all three versions in succession.

Workout 6
Kettlebell & Cardio

How it works
You'll be progressing through an ascending pyramid of row into kettlebell swing pairings. After a good warm-up, start at the first exercise and proceed up the exercise pyramid.

This workout starts off deceptively easy. In the early stages, you'll be thinking that you're going to get off lightly. But around the fourth row/swing pairing, you'll begin to feel the subtle physiological signs indicating an increase in exercise intensity. The knocking of your heart will grow louder. Sweat will pour more profusely from your brow. And a dull persistent ache will creep into your forearms, biceps, and shoulders. At this point the fight is on to the finish.

Methods of modification
If you're up to the challenge you can amplify the intensity of this kettlebell cardio workout by a) maintaining a high row pace (below 2:00/500 – that's 2-minutes per 500-metres), and/or b) going heavy on the kettlebell swings.

Of course, you don't have to stick with the exercises below. By way of example, a worthy substitute for rowing would be skipping. Instead of counting metres count skips. Though, if you did decide to skip, it would be wise to reduce the repetitions by half: 50 skips in place of 100-metre row.

As with the cardio exercise, you could replace the kettlebell swings for a comparable movement. If you didn't have access to a kettlebell, dumbbell thrusters would make an agreeable replacement.

Key points

- Concluding a progressive warm-up, begin at the first exercise – 100-metres row – and proceed to ascend the pyramid.
- Select the workout that reflects your current level of fitness.
- Aim to complete all sets unbroken.

Warm-up

- 2000-metre row – increase intensity every 500-metres
- Kettlebell swing pyramid: 1 up to 5 reps – then back down

Hungry4Fitness Kettlebell Cardio Workout			
Exercises	**Beginner**	**Intermediate**	**Advanced**
100m Row	2:30/500 row pace	2:00/500 row pace	1:55/500 row pace
10 Kettlebell Swings	8/16kg Kettlebell	16/24kg Kettlebell	24/40kg Kettlebell
200m Row	2:30/500 row pace	2:00/500 row pace	1:55/500 row pace
20 Kettlebell Swings	8/16kg Kettlebell	16/24kg Kettlebell	24/40kg Kettlebell
300m Row	2:30/500 row pace	2:00/500 row pace	1:55/500 row pace
30 Kettlebell Swings	8/16kg Kettlebell	16/24kg Kettlebell	24/40kg Kettlebell
400m Row	2:30/500 row pace	2:00/500 row pace	1:55/500 row pace
40 Kettlebell Swings	8/16kg Kettlebell	16/24kg Kettlebell	24/40kg Kettlebell

500m Row	2:30/500 row pace	2:00/500 row pace	1:55/500 row pace
50 Kettlebell Swings	8/16kg Kettlebell	16/24kg Kettlebell	24/40kg Kettlebell
600m Row	2:30/500 row pace	2:00/500 row pace	1:55/500 row pace
60 Kettlebell Swings	8/16kg Kettlebell	16/24kg Kettlebell	24/40kg Kettlebell
700m Row	2:30/500 row pace	2:00/500 row pace	1:55/500 row pace
70 Kettlebell Swings	8/16kg Kettlebell	16/24kg Kettlebell	24/40kg Kettlebell
800m Row	2:30/500 row pace	2:00/500 row pace	1:55/500 row pace
80 Kettlebell Swings	8/16kg Kettlebell	16/24kg Kettlebell	24/40kg Kettlebell
900m Row	2:30/500 row pace	2:00/500 row pace	1:55/500 row pace
90 Kettlebell Swings	8/16kg Kettlebell	16/24kg Kettlebell	24/40kg Kettlebell
1000m Row	2:30/500 row pace	2:00/500 row pace	1:55/500 row pace
100 Kettlebell Swings	8/16kg Kettlebell	16/24kg Kettlebell	24/40kg Kettlebell

Total metres rowed: 5500
Total kettlebell swings: 550

General advice

- Situate the rower and kettlebell as close together as possible. Ideally, you want to step off the rower and almost immediately be able to pick up the kettlebell.

This reduces wasted time when transitioning between kit and keeps the tempo ticking over.

- Use the first 100-metres of each row set to recover after the kettlebell swings. Do this instead of resting.

How it works

Each dumbbell exercise forms its own sub-workout. Organised into 'rounds', you are to complete 9 X 20-second high-intensity intervals. Concluding each individual 20-second round, you are to rest for the same duration.

Concluding the dumbbell HIIT, work through the cardio/callisthenic complex. All you're doing here is sprinting 50-metres then dropping straight into 25 reps of the accompanying body weight exercise. (The body weight exercises change with each sub-workout.) Remember, you don't have to stick to sprinting. Instead, you could, for example, row, cycle, or skip.

Once you've completed the first individual dumbbell HIIT, take a minute rest (if you absolutely must), then move to the next one in line.

Key points
- Complete each individual dumbbell HIIT.
- Once you have waded through the deluge of HIITs, have a bash at the cardio/calisthenics complex.

Warm-up
- Slow 50-metres jog followed by 5 press-ups, 5 air squats and 5 dumbbell thrusters (use a light pair of dumbbells). Repeat for 10-minutes ensuring to increase the intensity every 2-minutes or so. Max intensity over the last minute.

Workout

Dumbbell vertical lifts*

9 X 20-second rounds

5 X 50-metre sprint

5 X 25 reps squat thrusts

Dumbbell single-arm snatch

9 X 20-second rounds

5 X 50-metre sprint

5 X 25 reps air squat

Dumbbell squat jumps

9 X 20-second rounds

5 X 50-metre sprint

5 X 25 reps press-ups

Dumbbell thruster

9 X 20-second rounds

5 X 50-metre sprint

5 X 25 reps hanging leg raises (or 5 pull-ups)

General advice

- *The vertical lift, if you have yet to make acquaintance with this superb exercise, is simply a bicep curl into shoulder push press. Both dumbbells are curled then pressed at the same time.
- Prior to pulling your gloves on (metaphorically speaking) create a HIIT tracker so that you can chart progress through each dumbbell exercise. After completing a high-intensity interval, tick it off your tracker.
- Use a countdown timer when HIITing as this guarantees interval length accuracy while also facilitating training motivation.

How to hill sprint

First things first, to hill sprint you need a hill. Now, if you live in Norwich, Holland, or the Gobi Desert, you're going to struggle with this requirement. However, you can hill sprint on a treadmill. In fact, treadmills are better for hill sprint training because the gradient can be varied, and performance outputs more accurately measured.

When you've got a long straight stretch of road to run up, you're ready to start hill sprinting. The single more important part of a hill sprint workout is the warm-up. Warm-ups are an essential part of any training session. But, warming up is even more important when participating in high-intensity hill sprints for the fact that the gastrocnemius and Achilles tendon are placed under significant stress.

One simple way to ensure that you are thoroughly warm is to complete a low-intensity run, of between 2- to 3-miles, prior to your sprint workout. This confers a secondary benefit beyond preparing the calves and Achilles. By integrating a run into your hill sprint workout, you will make it a more inclusive training session.

Hill sprint methodology

Before arriving at the foot of the hill, you should have already determined how many sprint sets you are going to work through. Let's say that you plan to complete 10 X 50-metre sprints.

Unless you are trained and possess considerable fitness, it wouldn't be wise to attack the hill with the ferocity of Sisyphus; not for the first few sprints at least. If you start off at a high intensity you will likely fatigue early and fail to complete the sprint session.

Instead, organise and group the sprint sets into ascending intensities. Begin the workout at a low intensity building up to max over the latter sets. (See the hill sprint formulae below.)

How many hill sprints should I do?

The answer to that question hinges on two factors. First, your current level of fitness will largely determine how many hill sprints you can complete before you run out of steam.

A beginner might aim for three to five sprint sets with the goal of advancing the number of sets over time. For example, they could increase by one sprint every month until they reached 10 in total.

But that is only a suggestion. The beginner could decide to work through as many as 10 sprint sets. However, to get through the workout they would have to vary the intensity and take longer recovery periods.

The second factor has to do with your training goals. If you're just looking to mix things up a bit and/or want to improve general fitness, then one short hill sprint workout of three to five sets per week should be enough.

How long should the hill be for hill sprints?

A hill length of between 50- to 100-metres would more than suffice. Of course, it's not humanly possible to maintain maximum output for much more than 100-metres. Thus, a hill any longer is largely superfluous.

And because sprinting uphill is considerably more physically demanding than on a flat, few people could sustain a sprint beyond 50-metres before succumbing to fatigue.

Hill sprint workout

Before you begin the hill sprint workout in the table below, ensure to warm-up thoroughly first. I recommend tackling the 10 sprint sets after a slow 2- to 3-mile run. This approach will ensure that you are adequately prepared physiologically, but not overly fatigued that your performance will in any way be hindered.

As you have no doubt noticed, the intensity – percentage of max-effort – increases sharply across the three levels. Of course, beginners or the untrained are unlikely to sustain a high output for more than a couple of sets.

It's for this reason why the percentage of max-effort remains low through the early sets. The low intensity sets should be used as an additional warm-up and means of acclimatising to the coming demands of the session.

Remember, if you are a beginner, or your cardio is rust-ridden, reduce the number of sprints to suit your current level of fitness. There's absolutely no shame in amending the workout. You could start at two sets and increase by one (or two) each month.

Hungry4Fitness Hill Sprint Formulae			
Hill sprint sets	**Beginner**	**Intermediate**	**Advanced**
Set 1	40% max effort	50% max effort	60% max effort
Set 2	50% max effort	60% max effort	70% max effort
Set 3	50% max effort	60% max effort	80% max effort
Set 4	60% max effort	70% max effort	80% max effort

Set 5	60% max effort	70% max effort	90% max effort
Set 6	70% max effort	80% max effort	90% max effort
Set 7	70% max effort	80% max effort	90% max effort
Set 8	80% max effort	90% max effort	100% max effort
Set 9	50% max effort	100% max effort	100% max effort
Set 10	100% max effort	100% max effort	100% max effort

General advice

- Decide how many hill sprint sets you plan to complete *before* arriving at the foot of the hill.
- Begin your hill sprint workout at a low intensity and, on concluding each sprint, increase the intensity by 10%.

How it works

You can attack this barbell workout in a number of different ways. First, if your objective is to focus on strength development, you should aim for near-maximal lifts. After a good warm-up and a few light lifts, start packing on the poundage until you're in the strength training zone.

If you decide to go heavy ensure to observe strict form, aim for around six to 10 quality reps, and take plenty of rest between sets – 2- to 3-minutes. Also, if you plan to max out your final set, it's advisable to solicit the support of a spotter as this improves training safety. Moreover, a competent spotter can enable you to eke out more reps before you succumb to fatigue. This can greatly enhance strength gains.

But let's say that your aim is not purely about building strength. Perhaps you want to enhance muscular endurance as well. Concluding a rigorous warm-up and one or two practice sets, select a moderate weight, somewhere around 60 to 70% of maximum effort.

In contrast to the strength training protocol, aim for 10 to 15 good quality reps, for five to eight sets. Keep the rest periods short and try, if you can, to complete one full complex before stopping.

Barbell AMRAP

The final method you could have a go at is to treat this barbell-only workout as you would an AMRAP. Set yourself a countdown timer, of either five or 10-minutes, and try to accumulate as many repetitions as possible.

Of course, if you plan to have a bash at an AMRAP, it's advisable to select a weight that you can comfortably perform 10 reps with for all four exercises below. When AMRAPing, you want to avoid changing weight as it wastes precious time.

Key points
- Decide which training modality you plan to employ for this workout.
- Select a weight commensurate with your current strength and proceed through the workout.

Warm-up
1000-metres row or cross-trainer (or 5-minutes skipping)

1 X 250-metre cardio interval

10 reps deadlift (low resistance)

1 X 250-metre cardio interval

10 reps bent-over row

1 X 250-metre cardio interval

10 reps standing shoulder press

1 X 250-metre cardio interval

10 reps back squat

Workout
Deadlift
Option 1 strength training: 3 to 5 sets of 6 to 10 reps

Option 2 muscular endurance training: 5 to 7 sets of 12 to 20 reps

Option 3 AMRAP: set a 5-minute countdown timer and amass as many reps as your physicality will permit

Bent-over row
Option 1 strength training: 3 to 5 sets of 6 to 10 reps

Option 2 muscular endurance training: 5 to 7 sets of 12 to 20 reps

Option 3 AMRAP: set a 5-minute countdown timer and amass as many reps as your physicality will permit

Standing shoulder press
Option 1 strength training: 3 to 5 sets of 6 to 10 reps
Option 2 muscular endurance training: 5 to 7 sets of 12 to 20 reps
Option 3 AMRAP: set a 5-minute countdown timer and amass as many reps as your physicality will permit

Back squat
Option 1 strength training: 3 to 5 sets of 6 to 10 reps
Option 2 muscular endurance training: 5 to 7 sets of 12 to 20 reps
Option 3 AMRAP: set a 5-minute countdown timer and amass as many reps as your physicality will permit

---

General advice
- If your gig is strength augmentation, it's important to recruit the support of a spotter. Spotters not only help you to 'go heavy', but, more importantly, they improve training safety.
- If you're going to pit yourself against the AMRAP (rather you than me – 5-minutes of continuous squats? *Ouch!*) make a note of your rep scores. This will bequeath you with a benchmark to compete against if you ever pluck up the courage to have another go.

How it works

After you've warmed yourself by the fire of the mandatory warm-up, compose yourself mentally and then, starting from the first exercise, which is a 1000m run, work your way down to the 21st exercise as fast as you possibly can.

This workout could be completed at your local park. No equipment is needed save a patch of terra firma for the body weight exercises and a one-kilometre circuit to run around.

Key points

- Ensure that the warm-up is not included within the overall time.
- Complete all 21 exercises as fast as possible.
- Work through all exercises in the order shown.
- Stop the clock on completion of the very last metre of exercise 21.

Warm-up

1000-metre low intensity jog
50-metre sprint (60% max effort)
10 burpees
50-metre sprint (70% max effort)
10 burpees
50-metre sprint (80% max effort)
10 burpees
50-metre sprint (90% max effort)

10 burpees

50-metre sprint (100% max effort)

10 burpees

Workout

1. **1000m run**
2. 25 reps Burpees
3. 25 reps Press-ups
4. 50 reps Squat jumps
5. **1000m run**
6. 25 reps Burpees
7. 25 reps Press-ups
8. 50 reps Squat jumps
9. **1000m run**
10. 25 reps Burpees
11. 25 reps Press-ups
12. 50 reps Squat jumps
13. **1000m run**
14. 25 reps Burpees
15. 25 reps Press-ups
16. 50 reps Squat jumps
17. **1000m run**
18. 50 reps Burpees
19. 50 reps Press-ups
20. 100 reps Squat jumps
21. **1000m run**

General advice

- When performing the burpees make sure that you stand tall and jump at the top position.

- Try not to rest on completion of the exercises. Get straight back into the run!
- Do not lock the legs out at the top position of the squats.

Well Done
That's 10 Completed Workouts
Keep Going!

How it works

The objective here is to complete the six separate kettlebell swings into callisthenics circuits. You can either rest after each circuit or, if you want to challenge yourself, aim to work through them without pause.

If you opt for the latter approach, you might want to consider timing yourself. This will provide you with a standard to compete against the next time you undertake this workout.

Key points

- Complete each of the six separate kettlebell swing circuits.
- Either treat this as a conditioning workout or compete against the clock. If you opt for the former approach, ensure to enforce rest periods. If the latter, aim to complete the 300 reps in the shortest time possible.
- Concluding the kettlebell and callisthenic pairing, aim to go straight into the cardio blast.

Warm-up

- 2000-metre row
- 10 down to 1 pyramid of kettlebell swings and press-ups. If you're new to pyramiding the method is as follows: 10 reps swings/10 reps press-ups – then 9 reps swings/9 reps press-ups – etc., etc. Continue to descend the pyramid until you reach the final rep.

Workout

Circuit 1

➢ 25 reps Kettlebell swings
➢ 25 reps Squat jumps (challenge yourself by holding the kettlebell between your legs)
➢ 25 reps Kettlebell swings
➢ 25 reps Squat jumps
➢ 400-metre cardio blast (either run or row the distance)

Circuit 2

➢ 25 reps Kettlebell swings
➢ 25 reps Squat thrusts
➢ 25 reps Kettlebell swings
➢ 25 reps Squat thrusts
➢ 400-metre cardio blast

Circuit 3

➢ 25 reps Kettlebell swings
➢ 25 reps Burpees
➢ 25 reps Kettlebell swings
➢ 25 reps Burpees
➢ 400-metre cardio blast

Circuit 4

➢ 25 reps Kettlebell swings
➢ 25 reps Press-ups
➢ 25 reps Kettlebell swings
➢ 25 reps Press-ups
➢ 400-metre cardio blast

Circuit 5

➢ 25 reps Kettlebell swings

- ➤ 25 reps Triceps dips (full body weight if possible)
- ➤ 25 reps Kettlebell swings
- ➤ 25 reps Triceps dips
- ➤ 400-metre cardio blast

Circuit 6
- ➤ 25 reps Kettlebell swings
- ➤ 25 reps Pull-ups (full body weight if possible)
- ➤ 25 reps Kettlebell swings
- ➤ 25 reps Pull-ups
- ➤ 400-metre cardio blast

Totals
300 Kettlebell swings

300 Body weight reps

2400-metres ran/rowed

General advice
- Organise your equipment before embarking on the workout. This ensures an efficient transition between exercises.
- Aim to complete each circuit before resting.
- Consider timing yourself over the full circuit. When you are ready to have another crack at those 300 kettlebell swings, you'll have a time to compete against.

Workout 12
500 Kettlebell Swings

How it works

This workout is set out in a repeating circuit format (much the same as the one above). Comprised of three exercises – rowing, kettlebell swinging, and press-uping – your objective is to complete the triad before taking a rest. Of course, if you want to push yourself, or if you have the fitness, progress through the circuits without pause.

You'll notice that the row distances decrease by 250-metres with each successive circuit. Paradoxically, this makes the workout harder because you're afforded less time to rest between each set of 100 kettlebell swings. But remember, if you need to break the 100 kettlebell swings into smaller sets, say 50 or 25 reps, then you should do so.

The 25 press-ups serve a dual purpose in this workout. They engage the pectorals, possibly the one muscle group that swinging and rowing don't activate, and they help stretch off the forearms, which take a bit of beating from all that pulling and gripping.

Key points
- Focus on one step of the ascending exercise pyramid at a time.
- Aim to complete each step without resting.
- If you feel the need to split the kettlebell swings into sub-sets, do so!
- As advised in the 300 kettlebell swing workout, approach this as either conditioning or competition training. If you opt for the former take rests. If the latter, aim for the shortest time possible.

Warm-up

- 2000-metre row. After every 250-metres dismount the rower and complete 10 kettlebell swings.

Workout

- 1000-metre row
- 100 Kettlebell swings
- 25 Press-ups

- 750-metre row
- 100 Kettlebell swings
- 25 Press-ups

- 500-metre row
- 100 Kettlebell swings
- 25 Press-ups

- 250-metre row
- 100 Kettlebell swings
- 25 Press-ups

- 1000-metre row
- 100 Kettlebell swings
- 25 Press-ups

Totals

Distance rowed: 3500-metres

Kettlebell swings: 500

Press-ups: 125

General advice

- Organise your equipment before embarking on the workout.
- Consider timing yourself over the workout so that you have a benchmark to compete against the next time you have a go.

Workout 13
1300 Repetitions

How it works

You are to complete 100 repetitions on each exercise. Work through the circuit in the exact order laid out below – one down to 13. There's a catch with this session though. And that is, once you start an exercise you are forbidden from moving on *until* you have completed all one hundred reps.

Also, if you do rest between the 100 repetitions, regardless of how many times, you should perform a set of 10 burpees as a punishment. Example: if you split the bench press into sets of 25 reps you would incur 30 burpees: 25 reps bench press – 10 reps burpees – 25 reps bench press – 10 reps burpees – 25 reps bench press – 10 reps burpees – 25 reps bench press. Here you would have added 30 extra burpees to one exercise. Ouch!

With that in mind, I recommend that you rest as infrequently as possible between each exercise. (If this is a little too severe and you fear that you'll spend most of the circuit performing burpees, either a) scrap the punishment, or b) reduce punishment reps.)

Key points

- This is a lineal circuit which means that each exercise is visited only once.
- You are to perform 100 repetitions on each of the 13 exercises.
- Remember, if you need to break the 100 repetitions into smaller sub-sets, do so – just don't forget the burpee punishment!
- The resistance recommendations in parenthesis are exactly that, recommendations. You have complete carte blanche in selecting your own

weights. By way of caveat the only stipulation I would add is, ensure that the weight you select still presents a physical challenge.

Warm-up

- 2000m row
- Complete one lap of the circuit performing 10 repetitions on each exercise

Workout

1. 100 reps – Bench press (40kg)
2. 100 reps – Bent-over row (40kg)
3. 100 reps – Squats (40kg)
4. 100 reps – Hanging leg raises
5. 100 reps – Burpees
6. 100 reps – Press-ups
7. 100 reps – Lat pulldowns (40kg)
8. 100 reps – Squat thrusts
9. 100 reps – Step-ups (50 each leg) (2 X 10kg dumbbells)
10. 100 reps – Body weight squats (to 90-degree at the knee)
11. 100 reps – Kettlebell swing (24kg)
12. 100 reps – Kettlebell single-arm clean and jerk (50 each arm) (24kg)
13. 100 reps – Kettlebell squat (32kg)

General advice

- If you stop during an exercise, you should perform a set of 10 burpees.
- Throughout the step-ups and kettlebell clean and jerk, you are allowed to change to the opposite leg/arm as many times as you like.
- The bracketed resistances are suggestions only. Of course, depending on your strength, you can increase or decrease them accordingly.

Workout 14
10 X 2-Minute AMRAPs

How it works

Yes, this session requires kit and a bit of time spent setting it up, but I promise the payoff is well worth it. Once you're organised and ready to go, set a 2-minute countdown timer and attempt to complete as many repetitions/metres as you can on each of the 10 exercises.

The moment the 2-minute timer elapses make a note of your achievement and immediately advance to the following exercise. Hard though it is, resist the temptation to take a rest.

Follow on in this fashion until you have a score for all 10 exercises. (Next to each exercise, I have put my scores down to give you a benchmark to aim for.)

Key points

- Organise the equipment before starting the workout.
- Set a 2-minute countdown timer and attempt to amass as many repetitions and metres as possible before the buzzer sounds.
- Make a note of your scores so that you have a target to compete against next time.

Warm-up

- 10-minutes cardio and calisthenics – you decide the exercises. However, ensure to raise the intensity progressively across the duration of the warm-up.

Workout

1. 2-minutes kettlebell swings (28kg = 78 reps)

The kettlebell swing is a perfect whole-body exercise to kick this session into touch. Using the muscles of the posterior chain and core, propel the bell level with your shoulders. Try as best you can to maintain a continuous rhythm for the entirety of the 2-minutes.

2. 2-minutes ergo row (605-metres = 1:39/500 average)

Prior to disembarking fix your mind on a specific pace average and try to maintain it until the final 20-second sprint.

3. 2-minutes press-ups (76 reps)

You do not need to go lower than 90-degrees at the elbow. Adopt a hand position slightly over shoulder-width and, in sets of 5s or 10s, see how many sets you can complete before the sands of time drain dry.

4. 2-minutes Farmer's walk (2 x 34kg dumbbells – 200-metres)

Of course, before you started the session, you will have marked out and measured a runway. I placed two cones 20-metres apart and attempted to make as many crossings as possible. This tactic improves focus while also making calculating distance walked fuss-free.

5. 2-minutes double unders (122 jumps)

If you are not a competent skipper and you can't do double unders to save your eternal soul, simply perform single skips. However, remember that two single skips only count as one repetition.

6. 2-minutes vertical lifts (2 X 18kg dumbbells = 37 reps)

Holding a pair of dumbbells by your sides, you are to execute a biceps curl followed by a shoulder push press. A little tip: when curling the dumbbells up to the shoulders, generate a little swing then take a shallow dip at the knee and use your quadriceps to assist the second phase of the exercise.

7. 2-minutes medicine ball slams (8kg MB = 56 reps)

The medicine ball slam is such a brutish exercise. But it's brilliant for developing explosive power and muscular endurance. Initiating the movement with a deep sumo squat grasp the medicine ball and, hoisting it high above your head (like Atlas holding the world aloft), smash it into the floor with the ferocity of Thor bringing down his heavy hammer.

8. 2-minutes deadlifts (75kg = 35 reps)

For the second strength exercise of this session make sure that you take your time and apply near-perfect form: focus on quality over quantity. Adopting a slightly wider stance, a little over shoulder-width, grasp the bar.

Before executing a single rep ensure that your posture is prepared for the lift: back straight, core tight, looking forward. Set your sights on a specific rep count then, after each set, take a quick breather. Repeat for 120-seconds.

9. 2-minutes box jumps (one-metre box – 53 reps)

A plyometrics exercise par excellence, box jumps are a superlative dynamic leg-strength developer, and they also enhance explosive power to boot. In addition, they will hone timing, coordination, stamina, and mental discipline. Also, expect nasty DOMS in the lower abdominals a day or two after the workout.

Prior to performing plyometric box jumps just make sure that there are no dangerous objects nearby (apologies for the patronising egg suck, but you can never be too careful) and, if possible, place a cushioned mat by the box to absorb the impact.

10. 2-minute run on the treadmill at 10% incline (430-metres – 15kph average)

Before altering the speed first ensure that you have adjusted the incline to 10%. While the gradient is configuring, buckle up, blast the speed, and go supernova. This is the final exercise remember. So, you should use up any remaining juice left in the tank. And if you're all out? Well, run on fumes baby!

Cool-down

- 5-minutes of wallowing in a pool of sweat followed by a gentle walk on the treadmill

General advice

- Ensure to warm-up thoroughly before giving this workout a whirl.
- Be prepared for a tough physical fight. Granted, it's only a 20-minute workout. But you will be training at near-maximal intensity.

Workout 15
Cardio & Calisthenic Scorcher

This whole-body workout won't just sculpt visibly sharper muscles. The cute combination of cardiovascular and callisthenic exercises will also combust fat like naked flame to kerosine. Best to complete this session early in the week while willpower and motivation are high, and you're rested from a lazy weekend.

How it works

After polishing off the progressive warm-up you're going to be working through the 30 exercises as fast as possible. This is a 'lineal' circuit which means that you must start at the first exercise and then complete the proceeding 29 in the order shown.

The objective is to complete the circuit in the shortest time possible. So, as well as pushing yourself hard on each exercise, try to resist the temptation to rest between transitions.

Methods of modification

If necessity dictates, the cardio exercise can be substituted for any of the following alternatives: running, cycling, skipping – even swimming. Just make sure that the timings remain the same. By that I mean, if your average row speed is 2:00/500 (2-minutes per 500-metres), ensure to conduct the conversions for the cardio exercise substitute you select.

Key points
- Remain faithful to the exercise ordering.
- After setting a timer, progress through the 30 exercises as quickly as possible.
- Take the book with you to the gym and tick off the exercises as you go.

Warm-up

- 2000m row at a leisurely pace
- 1 up to 10 air squat and press-up pyramid. Methodology: 1 rep air squat followed by 1 rep press-up then straight into 2 reps air squats followed by 2 reps press-ups . . . finish on 10 reps each! (That's 110 total.)

Workout

1. **250m Row**
2. 50 Press-ups
3. **500m Row**
4. 50 Squat thrusts
5. 50 Squat jumps
6. 50 Burpees
7. **750m Row**
8. 50 Squat thrusts
9. 50 Squat jumps
10. 50 Burpees
11. **1000m Row**
12. 50 Squat thrusts
13. 50 Squat jumps
14. 50 Burpees
15. **1500m Row**
16. 50 Press-ups
17. 50 Squat thrusts
18. **2000m Row**
19. 50 Press-ups
20. 50 Squat jumps
21. **500m Row**
22. 50 Press-ups

23. 50 Squat jumps

24. 500m Row

25. 50 Press-ups

26. 1000k Row

27. 50 Air squats

28. 50 Squat thrusts

29. 50 Burpees

30. 2000m Row

Total reps = 1000

Total distance at speed = 10,000-metres

General advice

- Begin the workout at a moderate intensity.
- As you warm up to the workout, start pushing the tempo and aim to maintain a high intensity for as long as your physicality will permit.
- The final 2k row – post 50 burpees – is of course designed to push the limits of your aerobic fitness. Don't succumb to the temptation to take your foot off the accelerator and, please, whatever you do, don't quit!
- Finally, remember to stop the timer the moment you finish.

Workout 16
The Perfect Way to Start the Day

Richard Branson, billionaire entrepreneur and progenitor of the transnational conglomerate *Virgin*, purportedly said that an hour of exercise in the morning increases his productivity levels by four-hours. That's a hefty pay-off, more so considering the myriad health benefits associated with regular exercise.

While I'm yet to experience a four-hour bump in productivity levels, I agree that a morning workout is one of the best ways to start the day. Not only does an early sweat session wake you up to the world, but it starts the day on a healthy footing. And, as the saying goes, *start as you mean to go on.*

What I've found is that when I scrape myself out of bed and complete my obligatory morning workout routine (see below), I maintain healthy habits throughout the day, such as staying active, keeping hydrated, and abstaining from processed foods. Psychologically, it seems somewhat sacrilegious to subject yourself to sullying lifestyle practices after a cleansing cardio and calisthenics workout.

In addition to stoking the fires of self-discipline, I've also discovered that a morning training session promotes positive mental outlook. After completing the workout below, which is my standard 5 am morning routine, I'm typically much cheerier and thus embark on the day with a feel-good, can-do attitude.

And finally, I find that exercising first thing is energising. This at first may sound contradictory. After all, training is tiring – right? Though that seems logical, in my experience it's quite the opposite. A gentle 30- to 45-minute whole-body workout is like a battery boost, leaving me charged for the day ahead. So, with these benefits to be had, I invite you to join me on my morning routine.

How it works

On completion of the 10-minute warm-up, work through the five exercises below. The exercises have been organised into a circular circuit where one full lap typically takes 5-minutes. Most mornings I complete six laps which, including the warm-up and cool-down, equates to 45-minutes of training. However, if you don't have 45-minutes to spare in the morning, or you have recently resolved to embark on an exercise routine, simply cut the number of laps to suit your lifestyle requirements and current physical capacity.

Key points

- Warm-up with 10-minutes of gentle Yoga.
- When you feel awake, and your body stretched and loosened up, start the workout.

Warm-up

10-minutes Yoga

At 5 am every morning (except Sunday) I religiously roll out my Yoga mat and gently work through a series of sun salutations. The sun salutation, one of the 12 Basic Asanas of the Yogic Science, is a multifaceted movement 'that activates the myotatic stretch reflex' and, as well as increasing general flexibility, 'is especially good as a warm-up.'* From the sun salutation, I also perform a series of press-ups, plank, and air squats.

30-minutes cardio and calisthenics

Concluding Yoga, I jog to my local park where I complete a series of cardio and calisthenic circuits for 35-minutes. Because it's early and I'm still shrugging off the boon of sleep, I progress through the workout at a low- to moderate-intensity. As well as requiring no equipment, the following session is fully customisable. Meaning you change it however you please. But, if you do, just ensure that there is a cardio element and a series of functional body weight exercises.

Workout

1) 700-metre Run

Second to sun salutations running is the best morning exercise (in my opinion). A gentle jog helps clear the head as well as kickstart the heart and open the lungs. In addition, running is a great fat burner and whole-body fitness developer. During this morning workout, I take it nice and easy and maintain a plodding pace for the first couple of laps.

2) 25 reps Hanging leg raises

HLRs are more than merely an abdominal toner. They develop core stability and grip strength. Furthermore, they are eminently modifiable – meaning you can either settle for easy knee raises or test yourself with toes to bar. And if HLRs ever get too easy, which they never do, there's always the option of increasing the resistance by gripping a weight between your knees.

3) 25 reps Alternate leg squat thrusts

A highly functional movement, alternate leg squat thrusts train multiple muscle groups. This is because they are an amalgamation of two exercises. While holding the high plank position (the start of a press-up) you are to pump your legs back and forward like a pair of pistons. As well as engaging your cardiovascular system, they'll build stamina and muscle endurance in the arms, chest, abdominals, and glutes.

4) 25 reps Press-ups

Press-ups are revered for their fitness-developing and body-sculpting qualities. They are brilliant at building pectoral, anterior deltoid, and triceps strength. Furthermore, they work the transverse abdominus, abdominal muscles, and hip flexors. Also, the press-ups are eminently modifiable and there are (apparently) over 25 different variations.

5) 25 reps Air squats

The air squat is a simple yet effective exercise for developing muscle endurance in the quadriceps. They are perfect for a morning workout for two reasons. First, they are low intensity. Second, because you're only squatting two-thirds of your total body weight, air squats do not over-stress the leg joints. However, once I've warmed up after a couple of laps of the circuit, I add a plyometric jump onto the squat which quickly intensifies this relatively easy exercise.

Cool-down

As a nice treat (and to cool-down) I'll enjoy a 5-minute walk home where, after a shower, I'll cook a healthy breakfast: porridge (water and not bovine lactate) topped with seeds, crushed nuts, fresh berries, and perhaps a drizzle of natural honey.

General advice

- Aim to use this workout as your weekly morning wake-up session.
- Start off nice and slow and take your time through the exercises.
- Do not put any pressure on yourself to complete every aspect of the workout. Some days, when I'm not feeling the love, as it were, I just go for a gentle morning walk and pay the park a visit where I'll perform a calisthenics complex.
- *The supporting citation solicited to substantiate the merit and worth of the sun salutation was taken from Herbert David Coulter's brilliant book *Anatomy of Hatha Yoga*.

Workout 17
The Ultimate Sandbag Session

Before we begin, it's probably worth clarifying what sandbag training is, in case you are unfamiliar with this contemporary exercise tool. Sandbags are in many respects similar to powerbags. The primary difference is that, unlike powerbags, sandbags are not fashioned from a rigid material. Meaning the weight moves about which makes it more challenging to control.

This may not initially sound like an attribute worthy of commendation, but it is. Why? Well, quite simply because to control the sandbag, to hoist it into position and hold it securely, you are required to engage a wider range of muscle groups. It's this quality of sandbags that make them excellent for developing functional strength.

How it works

Concluding the warm-up, you are to work through the five sandbag pyramids. Starting at the foot of the first pyramid, you will perform one repetition then complete a 100-metre sprint. Slowly jog back to the sandbag and now perform two repetitions.

As soon as you've completed your reps jump straight into the sprint. Repeat until you have progressed up to the 10th repetition. At this point you could take a rest or get straight into the next exercise pyramid.

Method of modification

This sandbag workout is fully modifiable. For example, you could replace the run with any other cardiovascular exercise. Skipping or rowing are great substitutes for running if you're not a fan.

Furthermore, if the training volume is too high for your current level of fitness, simply reduce the pyramids by half. And if you've yet to buy a sandbag? Simply substitute it with a different item of training equipment – a powerbag or kettlebell would work well – or perform body weight exercises.

Another simple way of modifying this workout is by reducing (or increasing!) the sprint lengths. They are set at 100-metres. However, that distance is not etched in stone. You could reduce it to 50-metres or even 25-metres.

Key points

- Warm-up well before attempting this workout.
- Progress up the pyramid ensuring to perform the post-sandbag sprints.
- Work through each pyramid as fast as your physicality will permit.
- Aim to complete all five pyramids without resting. But if you do need to pause for a breather, set a 30-second countdown timer and rigidly stick to the temporal stipulation.

Warm-up

- 10-minutes of light jogging and calisthenics. Slowly jog 100-metres (or thereabouts) and complete one press-up. Jog back the perform two press-ups. Repeat until you reach five press-ups. Now change the exercise.

Workout

1: Sandbag bent-over rows

Bent-over rows are one of the best upper-body strength-building exercises. They are unparalleled for developing back and arm pulling power. Sandbag bent-over rows are performed the same as the barbell version.

1 rep	2 reps	3 reps	4 reps	5 reps	6 reps	7 reps	8 reps	9 reps	10 reps
100m	100m	100m	100m	100m	100m	100m	100m	100m	100m

2: Sandbag squats

If you want strong legs and cut quads, then you can't keep avoiding squats. Sandbag squats offer a lighter alternative for those who don't enjoy this brutish exercise. But if they start to get too easy, you always have the option of adding an explosive plyometric jump.

1 rep	2 reps	3 reps	4 reps	5 reps	6 reps	7 reps	8 reps	9 reps	10 reps
100m	100m	100m	100m	100m	100m	100m	100m	100m	100m

3: Sandbag hang cleans

The hang clean is an excellent hip extension developer. And strong hip extension translates to improved performance across a range of fitness and sporting disciplines. Sandbag hang cleans are performed the same way as the barbell version.

1 rep	2 reps	3 reps	4 reps	5 reps	6 reps	7 reps	8 reps	9 reps	10 reps
100m	100m	100m	100m	100m	100m	100m	100m	100m	100m

4: Sandbag lunge to side twist

You've got to remain focused when performing sandbag lunge to side twists. If you're thinking about what's for dinner or what's on Netflix, you'll wind up losing balance and potentially your footing. Remember to step to the side as you step forward as this creates a stable base.

1 rep	2 reps	3 reps	4 reps	5 reps	6 reps	7 reps	8 reps	9 reps	10 reps
100m	100m	100m	100m	100m	100m	100m	100m	100m	100m

5: Sandbag hang cleans to overhead heaves

The final exercise is an extension of the third. After performing the hang clean explosively heave the sandbag over your head. To take this exercise to another dimension perform a burpee into press-up (aka a bastod) prior to the hang clean.

1 rep	2 reps	3 reps	4 reps	5 reps	6 reps	7 reps	8 reps	9 reps	10 reps
100m	100m	100m	100m	100m	100m	100m	100m	100m	100m

General advice

- Do not worry so much about trying to maintain perfect form when executing the sandbag lifts. I know that's a heretical statement coming from an exercise and fitness professional (self-styled). But sandbag training is supposed to be functional. Thus, it's more emulative of real life: we don't ensure perfect spinal alignment when heaving the shopping into the car boot or squatting on and off the throne.
- The idea is to handle the sandbag like a nightclub bouncer would a boozed-up belligerent. Get rough, get ready, get physical!

How it works

There are two ways you can approach this dumbbell leg workout. This first is to apply the age-old sets/reps/rest method. For each of the five exercises complete the specified number of repetitions for the stipulated number of sets. Concluding each set take a 30-second rest.

The second method has a CrossFit flavour to it; making it much more intense. Comprised of five individual AMRAPs, you are to set a 5-minute countdown on your training timer. As soon as the timer starts you are to perform as many repetitions as possible inside the allotted time. Make a note of your score so that you have something to compete against next time you try this leg workout.

Methods of modification

Because dumbbells are a super-versatile training tool you can swop and change any of the exercises below for ones that suit your preferences. If you choose to do this just ensure to follow the routine as closely as possible.

While working through the first approach method (see above) you could, instead of resting, complete upper body exercises. By incorporating upper body exercises into this workout, you would make it a complete training session.

Let's say you decided to have a go at the second approach method, the five AMRAPs, but you felt that your fitness wasn't quite up to the challenge. Don't be deterred. Instead, reduce the AMRAP duration from 5-minutes to 3-minutes. Even by lowering the duration to 3-minutes, you'd still get a damn good workout. Also, starting below the stipulated duration will provide you with a fitness goal to pursue. Every time you have a bash at this workout, increase the AMRAP duration by one-minute until you hit your target.

Key points

- Before embarking on this leg builder, decide which approach method you plan to apply.
- Don't forget to warm-up.
- Accompanied only by a pair of dumbbells, sequester yourself away from the general gym population and proceed to progress through the following five exercises.

Warm-up

- 5k cycle on the stationary bike. Starting at resistance 10, increase by 2 every kilometre.
- Concluding the cycle, complete a 1 up to 10 and then 10 down 1 ascending and descending squat jump pyramid. The *burn!*
- 2k cycle – set the resistance low but maintain a high cadence (90 to 100 RPM).

Workout

1: Bulgarian split squat
First approach
Reps: 10 each side
Sets: 3 to 5
Rest: 60-seconds

Second approach
5-minute AMRAP: to balance the workload it is advisable to switch legs after each rep. How many reps can you perform?

Bulgarian split squat teaching points
- Rest the instep of your back foot on a stable object – such as a training bench or chair – and plant your front foot so it's facing forwards. The start position should resemble a shallow lunge.
- Ensure that your hips and shoulders are facing forwards; your torso should be vertical.
- Keeping your core contracted throughout, lower under control until the quad of your active leg is parallel to the floor.
- At no point during this exercise should the toes of your lunging leg disappear behind your knee. If they do, you need to readjust your position so that your foot is further away from the bench.

2: Side lunge
First approach
Reps: 10 each side
Sets: 3 to 5
Rest: 60-seconds

Second approach
5-minute AMRAP: alternating between each leg how many reps can you perform?

Side lunge teaching points
- Holding a pair of dumbbells at your sides, stand with your feet close together, toes pointing forward.
- Take a double shoulder-width step to the side and execute a lunge onto your leading leg.
- To enhance the movement, bend your leading knee until the dumbbells touch either side of your foot. If you've got the strength and flexibility, you could even touch the floor.
- To complete the repetition fire through the quadriceps explosively until you are standing back in the start position.
- Repeat on the opposite leg.

3: Sumo squat
First approach
Reps: 10 each side
Sets: 3 to 5
Rest: 60-seconds

Second approach
5-minute AMRAP: alternating between each leg how many reps can you perform?

Sumo squat teaching points
- With a pair of dumbbells positioned at your feet, adopt a double shoulder-width stance – as a Sumo wrestler would – toes pointing forward, torso nice and straight.
- Squat down grasp the dumbbells and stand back up.
- You are now in the start position and ready to perform a sumo squat.
- With the dumbbells dangling between your legs execute a squat ensuring to follow the same protocol as you would when performing a barbell squat.
- Keep your knees in line with your toes throughout.
- Your back is perfectly straight.
- Synchronise your breathing with the concentric and eccentric contraction phases of the exercise.
- If you're up for a nasty burn in the quad explode out of the squat into a plyometric jump.

4: Reverse lunge
First approach
Reps: 10 each side
Sets: 3 to 5
Rest: 60-seconds

Second approach
5-minute AMRAP: alternating between each leg how many reps can you perform?

Reverse lunge teaching points
- The start position of the reverse lunge is the same as the forward lunge: feet slightly apart; back upright; dumbbells by your sides.
- Now, as the name suggests, step back into a lunge ensuring to bend your leading leg. Do not make the common mistake of touching the floor with your knee. This could injure your patella.
- As you smoothly sink into the reverse lunge maintain correct postural alignment: dumbbells by your sides; shoulders braced; back straight; looking forward not down.
- To return to the start position power out of the lunge from the *rear*.

5: Dumbbell step-up
First approach
Reps: 10 each side
Sets: 3 to 5
Rest: 60-seconds

Second approach
5-minute AMRAP: alternating between each leg how many reps can you perform?

Dumbbell step-up teaching points
- To perform this exercise, you will need a stable object on which to step. I advise against antique furniture and the side of your sofa. If you have a plyometrics box, use that. The box or stable object should be about the height of your knee. (If you want to increase the intensity increase the height of the box.)
- With an ironing board-straight back and grasping two dumbbells by your sides, proceed to step up onto the box.
- Ensure to plant your *full* foot on the box and not just your toes. This makes the exercise a little bit harder but a lot safer.
- To conclude the repetition, step back down under control.
- When your leading foot is planted on the floor initiate the next repetition ensuring to observe all the preceding teaching points.

General advice

- Before attempting the workout ensure that you are thoroughly familiarised with the dumbbell exercises. I say this because in all likelihood you haven't performed Bulgarian split squats before. No probs. Read over the tutorial and have a go with a light pair of DBs. If you're more of a visual learner, punch the exercise into YouTube and watch one of the trillion tutorials.

Workout 19
30-Minute Barbell Complex

How it works

Comprised of six exercises, your objective is to work through them following the order laid out below. However, there are three different training approaches (options) that you can choose from.

Option 1: Traditional barbell workout

Option one is based on a traditional weightlifting method. You're going to complete three to five sets of between six to 12 reps. Sticking as closely as you can to the traditional method, begin your first set with a lighter load and increase the resistance as you decrease the reps.

If you plan to push the poundage, ensure to take plenty of rest between sets. You need to allow those muscles time to recover so that you can squeeze every last drop of strength out of them.

Option 2: AMRAP

The second method is considerably more demanding and is for those who fancy a tough physical challenge. The objective here is quite simple.

For 5-minutes you are to perform as many reps as possible on each of the six exercises. Set a countdown timer and rep-out until your muscles burst into flame.

You can of course take a rest during an AMRAP. But if you do succumb to the temptation to rest, ensure to keep it short. Every second lost is a missed opportunity to eke out another rep.

Option 3: EMOM

The third and final option is based on the CrossFit training method called EMOM – which is an acronym for *every minute on the minute*.

Each barbell exercise is comprised of five one-minute 'rounds.' The objective is to complete the set number of repetitions inside one-minute. Once you have completed the repetitions, you can rest for however many seconds remain on the countdown timer.

Remember, the second the minute elapses, you must begin the next set without a moment's delay. When you have completed all five one-minute rounds, progress to the next barbell exercise.

Key points
- Decide which of the three workout options you plan to tackle.
- Grab yourself an Olympic barbell, a pair of clips, an assortment of weight plates, and have yourself a fitness feast!

Warm-up
- 5-minute steady-paced row. Aim to increase the intensity every minute.
- Concluding the initial phase, complete 10 X 100-metre sprints followed by 10 repetitions of the barbell exercises in the workout.
- Only select one barbell exercise per sprint and change the exercises as you progress through the 10 intervals.

Workout
Standing shoulder press
Option 1: 3 to 5 sets of 6 to 12 repetitions.
Option 2: 5-minute AMRAP – how many reps did you achieve?

Option 3: 5-minute EMOM – aim for between 8 and 16 reps on the minute every minute.

Standing shoulder press teaching points
- Stand with feet shoulder-width apart, knees bent, with an Olympic barbell suspended level with your shoulders.
- The bar should be slightly below your chin or just above your shoulders
- Maintaining control, press the barbell above your head.
- At 'full extension' there should still be a slight bend at the elbow joints.
- To conclude the press, lower the barbell back to the start position.

Bicep curl
Option 1: 3 to 5 sets of 6 to 12 repetitions.
Option 2: 5-minute AMRAP – how many reps did you achieve?
Option 3: 5-minute EMOM – aim for between 16 and 24 reps on the minute every minute.

Bicep curl teaching points
- Gripping an Olympic bar at your front, palms facing out, position your feet shoulder-width apart. The knees are slightly bent.
- An Olympic barbell positioned in front of your quadriceps.
- In a controlled movement curl the barbell until it is level with your anterior deltoid.
- Remember, as you curl the barbell, concentrate on applying equal force through both biceps.
- After a quick 'squeeze' at the point of peak contraction, return the barbell back to the start position.

Bench press
Option 1: 3 to 5 sets of 6 to 12 repetitions.
Option 2: 5-minute AMRAP – how many reps did you achieve?

Option 3: 5-minute EMOM – aim for between 12 and 20 reps on the minute every minute.

Bench press teaching points
- Lie back on a flat bench, feet planted firmly on the floor, spaced a little over shoulder-width, a barbell positioned level with your chest.
- If you're in the correct position the bar should be directly over your nips, your hands spaced 1.5 shoulder-widths and a slight kink in the elbow joints.
- Keeping your eyes fixed on a point on the ceiling, lower the barbell under control until it gently touches your chest.
- Do not hold your breath during the exercise.
- Try, if you can, to synchronise your breathing with the eccentric and concentric contraction phases of the movement: breathe in as you lower the bar and out as your press the bar.
- Keep control throughout and focus on executing flawless form.

Bent-over barbell row
Option 1: 3 to 5 sets of 6 to 12 repetitions.
Option 2: 5-minute AMRAP – how many reps did you achieve?
Option 3: 5-minute EMOM – aim for between 12 and 20 reps on the minute every minute.

Bent-over barbell row teaching points
- Adopt a neutral stance: feet shoulder-width; knees slightly bent; eyes fixed forward.
- The barbell should be resting in front of your quadriceps, your hands spaced shoulder-width, palms facing inwards.
- Hinging at the hips only, lower until the barbell is level with your knees.
- Your back should be perfectly straight, and you should still be looking forward.
- In one smooth movement row the barbell to your lower abdomen.
- The elbows, when rowing, should not protrude to the side. Also, avoid 'cocking' the wrists.

Barbell deadlift

Option 1: 3 to 5 sets of 6 to 12 repetitions.

Option 2: 5-minute AMRAP – how many reps did you achieve?

Option 3: 5-minute EMOM – aim for between 6 and 10 reps on the minute every minute.

Barbell deadlift teaching points

- Start with your feet under the Olympic barbell adopting a stance slightly over shoulder-width.
- Bending at the knee and ensuring to keep the back perfectly straight, grasp the bar.
- The palms should face toward you and your hands should be spaced slightly wider than your feet to prevent your arms and knees clashing.
- Before executing the lift take the slack out of the bar by applying force against the resistance.
- Looking forward and slightly up fire through the quads and glutes pushing the hips forwards as you stand.
- Once you are fully erect there should be a slight bend in the knees – not locked out.
- Also, from a side angle, a vertical line could be drawn from your shoulders through your hips down to your heels.
- A common mistake is to lean back. **DO NOT** do this! All you will succeed in doing is compressing the intervertebral discs in the lumbar region.
- To conclude the exercise simply return the bar to the start position making sure to retrace your steps.
- To make deadlifting safer, use bumper plates so that you can drop the bar.

Barbell squat

Option 1: 3 to 5 sets of 6 to 12 repetitions.

Option 2: 5-minute AMRAP – how many reps did you achieve?

Option 3: 5-minute EMOM – aim for between 8 and 16 reps on the minute every minute.

Barbell squat teaching points

- With an Olympic barbell resting across your trapezius, adopt a slightly wider stance – just over shoulder-width.
- Your knees are bent and you are looking forward.
- Slowly and under control squat down until a 90-degree angle forms behind the knee.
- Again, maintaining strict form stand up out of the squat.
- Remember to apply equal force through both quadriceps.
- Also, do not hinge at the hips or round the back at any point throughout the movement.

General advice

- Ensure to warm-up thoroughly prior to progressing through this barbell complex.
- Select a weight that is commensurate with your current level of strength.
- It's worth having a few spare weight plates lingering about the place for when you want to turn up the temperature. Of course, a weight that'll cause your biceps to pop won't even make your quads quiver.

How it works

The structure of this workout couldn't be simpler. Your objective is to complete 10 repetitions on each of the eight kettlebell exercises, which are organised into a single circuit.

On completion of one circuit, you are to attack the cardio and calisthenics complex. This consists of short shuttle sprints interspersed with a descending body weight exercise pyramid.

So, after sprinting 25-metres, you will drop straight down and polish off 10 burpees. From the burpees, you're straight back into another 25-metre sprint but this time followed by eight burpees. Continue in this fashion until you complete two burpees. That constitutes as one 'round'.

After subjecting your heart to multiple sprint-into-burpee slaps get straight back into the next kettlebell circuit. Repeat for a minimum of five full rounds. Real fitness warriors settle for no fewer than 10 rounds on the bounce!

Key points

- Select a challenging kettlebell weight. If, for example, you can comfortably lift 16kg (1-pood), have a bash at 24kg (1.5-poods). But keep that 16kg close by just in case you can't handle that additional half pood.
- The eight kettlebell exercises are to be completed in the order shown. Do not deviate from the plan!

- You should aim to progress smoothly through the eight exercises without downing your bell. I ought to have imposed a 25-burpee punishment for bell downing – such a heinous crime! Maybe next time.

Warm-up

- 10-minute skipping followed by 10 X 25 skip sprints into 10 reps kettlebell swings

Workout

1: Kettlebell swings – 10 reps

- Hold the kettlebell between your legs, palms facing inwards, feet a little over shoulder-width apart.
- Pull the bell back and, using your glutes, propel it forward and up level with your shoulders.
- Ensuring to keep your core engaged throughout the movement, allow the kettlebell to return to the start position and repeat.

2: Kettlebell squats – 10 reps

- Adopt the same position as above: kettlebell between your legs, palms facing inwards, feet spaced slightly over shoulder-width apart.
- Fix your eyes forward and, keeping a straight back, bend at the knee.
- When your knees reach 90-degrees pause and return to the start position. Remember: don't lock your knees at the top.

3: Single-arm cleans – 10 reps (5 each arm)

- Adopting a shoulder-width stance (or slightly wider), grasp the kettlebell.
- In one fluid movement swing it back between your legs.
- Fire the bell forward using glute strength.
- Cutting the trajectory short, pull the bell into the nook of the arm.
- Pause then return and repeat.

4: Single-arm jerk – 10 reps (5 each arm)

- To get the kettlebell into position perform the first phase of the clean.
- Taking a shallow dip at the knees, use your quadriceps to generate a bit of momentum in the kettlebell.
- Assist the upward flight of the kettlebell with shoulder and arm strength.
- Take a second dip at the knees while simultaneously locking the arm out. Stand up as you do so.
- From here return the kettlebell back to the nook of the arm.
- Pause monetarily before performing the next jerk.

5: Under the leg pass – 10 passes

- Standing over the kettlebell space your feet about 1.5 shoulder-widths. The knees remain bent.
- Grasp the kettlebell and straighten the knees a touch. The kettlebell should now be suspended a foot off the floor and your knees still slightly bent.
- Keeping the back straight and flexing at the hips, proceed to 'thread' or 'weave' the bell back behind and through your legs.
- Now continue to trace out a figure of eight.

6: Single-arm snatch – 10 reps (5 each arm)

- Stand over the kettlebell adopting a shoulder-width stance.
- Flexing at the hips grasp the kettlebell and pull it back between your legs.
- Using glute strength propel the bell forward. You need to apply a lot of *humph!* to get it going.
- Guide the bell high above your head using your core and shoulder muscles.
- Arrest the bell directly above your head.
- There should be a slight bend at the elbow of the supporting arm. The other can be held out to the side for balance and stability.
- Allowing gravity to do the work, let the kettlebell drop into the original start position.
- However, do not slow or impede its momentum. For this should be harnessed for the next rep.

7: Kettlebell deadlifts – 10 reps

- Hold the kettlebell in front of your thighs, with palms facing inwards and your legs shoulder-width apart.
- Hinge at the hips and, keeping your hamstrings straight, scrape the kettlebell down your inner calves.
- Engage your core and bring your chest parallel with the floor before completing the exercise.

8: Kettlebell thruster – 10 reps

- Standing over the kettlebell, take a reverse grip of the handle.
- In one clean movement upturn the kettlebell and hold it out in front of your chest.
- In the start position, your arms form perfect right-angles, and the base of the kettlebell should be facing the ceiling.
- Keeping your back straight squat to 90-degrees, or until your forearms touch the top of your quads.
- Power out of the squat ensuring, as you do so, to push the kettlebell high above your head.
- From the outstretched position lower the kettlebell back to your chest while simultaneously sinking into the next squat.

Cardio/calisthenics pyramid

25-metre shuttle sprint – 10 burpees
25-metre shuttle sprint – 8 burpees
25-metre shuttle sprint – 6 burpees
25-metre shuttle sprint – 4 burpees
25-metre shuttle sprint – 2 burpees

General advice

- Prior to picking up that kettlebell make sure that you can perform all the exercises with the technical proficiency of a seasoned girevik. If your technique is anything less than exemplary (safe will do), spend a week polishing and perfecting your kettlebell handling skills before having a go at this workout. When you're a master of sport, come back and give it hell!

- If the only access you have to a kettlebell is at your gym, substitute the sprints for skipping. This way you won't have to bother with getting on and off the treadmill to complete the cardio/calisthenics pyramid.

Well Done
That's 20 Completed Workouts
Keep Going!

Workout 21
Buy One Get Two Free

The three outdoor workouts below have been designed to develop functional strength, facilitate fat loss, and improve whole-body fitness. In addition, because the workouts contain a cardiovascular element – either jogging, sprints and/or hill sprints – they will also improve your aerobic capacity. Thus, if you regularly participate in these outdoor workouts, you should enjoy a plethora of positive physiological outcomes.

It's this combination of cardio and calisthenics that makes these three outdoor workouts ideal for conditioning training. The body weight exercises develop muscle definition and physical functionality, while the cardio exercises facilitate fat loss and the augmentation of aerobic fitness.

Furthermore, because these outdoor workouts don't require a single item of exercise equipment, they can be completed almost anywhere. This means that, if for whatever reason you cannot access a gym, you'll always have a whole-body training session to hand.

Key points
- A **How it works** explanation can be found under the title of each of the three workouts. But the key points are as follows:
- Concluding the warm-up, which is typically integrated into the main session, progress through the workout of your choosing.
- The duration and exercise volume both increase with each successive workout.
- The workouts have not been crafted to meet variations in fitness levels. Thus, irrespective of your current physical capability, you can have a go at whichever

workout tickles your pickle. However, in saying that, if you focus on each workout for a week, you'll have nearly a month of exercise entertainment. You're welcome!

30-Minute workout

The following training session is one of my personal favourites and it is my go-to Sunday morning routine. It has been designed to develop muscular endurance and cardiovascular fitness. Here's how I approach this workout.

Just up the road from my house is a park around which skirts a perimeter path. The path has been marked out with posts spaced 100 metres apart. There are seven posts. At one end of the park is an area where exercises can be performed. This is the circuit that I've tailored to this urban environment:

Warm-up (5/10-minutes) (walking/jogging/body-weight exercises)

- 1 x lap of the park (700-metres)
- 25 reps Burpees
- 25 reps Press-ups
- 25 reps Squat jumps
- 25-seconds Plank
- 5 reps Pull-ups

Repeat 5 times

Each full lap, including the 100 reps, takes roughly 6-minutes – at a leisurely Sunday morning pace. The structure of this session makes it perfect for the person who is time-constrained or has recently started out on their physical training journey. For not only can the resistance exercises be interchanged with ones more preferable, but the number of laps can be tailored to suit your pre-budgeted training time or current fitness level.

45-Minute workout

Whereas the distances and repetitions of the first session are split across a series of sets (or circuits), session two focuses on each component separately. That is, complete the run distance (or cardiovascular exercise) then work through a series of body weight exercises.

- 30-minute jog
- 15-minute AMRAP
- 10 reps Press-ups
- 10 reps Step-ups
- 10 reps Triceps dips (either full body weight or partial)
- 10 reps Burpees

After the run – which serves as an extended warm-up – the aim here is to complete as many repetitions as possible (AMRAP) in 15-minutes. Once you've set your timer, start at the first exercise, and proceed to work through them in the order shown. Try not to rest for the duration of the AMRAP and ensure that you make a note of how many cycles you have completed.

1-Hour workout

Session three starts with a 30-minute jog. (Feel free to substitute running for a different cardiovascular exercise such as cycling, skipping, or rowing.) Following the run, you will complete a series of calisthenics pyramids coupled with sprints.

After completing the first level of the pyramid, you are to sprint 50/75/100-metres (select distance appropriate to your level of fitness). The objective here is to initiate the sprint straight out of the set of press-ups.

The moment you have completed the sprint either jog or walk back to the area where you are performing the callisthenic exercises. This constitutes as your recovery time. On returning, drop down immediately into the next set. Repeat until you have progressed up the pyramid. Proceed in this fashion through the four exercises.

- 30-minute run
- 1 up to 10 press-ups
- 1 up to 10 squats
- 1 up to 10 plank (reps are replaced with seconds: 5 reps = 5-seconds)
- 1 up to 10 burpees

General advice

- If you're untrained or new to this type of training, set your sights on completing the 30-minute workout. When you get a feel for the mechanics and physical demands, move on.
- Of course, because these workouts are completed independently of a gym, you are restricted to the resistance of your body weight. This is a recognised limitation of the workouts. However, to circumvent this minor problem, purchase a resistance band and take it with you to the park. Resistance bands, as well as being inexpensive and eminently portable, are a dynamic way to increase the resistance of body weight exercises.

Workout 22
Military Combat Training

This workout is inspired by battle-fitness training I used to do as a Royal Marines Commando. But don't worry, it doesn't involve guns, explosives, or sadomasochistic Physical Training Instructors.

How it works

First, you're going to warm-up with a gentle 2.5-mile jog. Maintaining a steady pace, this distance should take no longer than 20-minutes. Concluding the run, you are to work through the four sprint-to-body weight exercise AMRAPs below. Let me just quickly take a minute out of your day to explain how to approach these AMRAPs.

You need to mark out a 50-metre stretch of flat ground, preferably a path at your local park or, better still, a patch of grass. (If you really want to push yourself, find a hill to sprint up!) Then set a 5-minute countdown timer.

As soon as the clock starts you are to sprint the 50-metre distance. The moment you pass the line drop down and complete 10 repetitions of the stipulated body weight exercise. Repeat for 5-minutes! Nasty I know. But then this workout is supposed to simulate military combat training.

After the buzzer sounds signifying the end of the 5-minute AMRAP, enjoy a well-deserved one-minute rest. Is that all! One measly minute? Yep, that's your lot soldier! Okay, now that you are adequately rested and, no doubt, raring to get stuck into the next AMRAP, again start the countdown timer for round two. Repeat this heart-palpitating procedure until you have progressed through the four 5-minute AMRAPs.

Key points

- Concluding the progressive 10-minute warm-up, compose yourself both mentally and physically, then attack the 2.5-mile run.
- Aim to sustain a pace around 70 to 80% of your maximum effort. When you finish the run, you should be suffering.
- Following hot on the heels of the run are the four sprints into calisthenics AMRAPs.
- Apply a similar work ethic throughout the AMRAPs as with the run: maintain 70 to 80% max effort.

Warm-up

- 10-minute jogging: walk for a couple of minutes before breaking into a slow jog. Progressively increase the tempo until you have reached that pace which you plan to maintain for the 2.5-mile run.

Workout

- 2.5-mile run (aim to complete in under 20-minutes)

- 5-minute AMRAP 1: 50-metre sprint followed by 10 press-ups
- **1-minute rest**

- 5-minute AMRAP 2: 50-metre sprint followed by 10 star jumps
- **1-minute rest**

- 5-minute AMRAP 3: 50-metre sprint followed by 10 burpees
- **1-minute rest**

- 5-minute AMRAP 4: 50-metre sprint followed by 10 bastods (burpee with a press-up)

General advice

- Warm-up well before the run. Contrary to common misunderstanding, warming up prior to exercise does not drain our supply of energy. Quite the opposite in fact. A progressive pre-workout warm-up has been shown to improve physical performance as well as fanning the flames of training motivation.
- I know you're sick of hearing my say this but consider keeping track of your performance through each AMRAP. That is, tallying how many sprints you achieved in 5-minutes. This way you'll have a benchmark to compete against if you ever pluck up the courage to have another go at this workout in the future.
- If you can't find a suitable patch of ground to complete the AMRAP sprints, you can skip instead (50 skips = 50-metres).

Workout 23
21 CrossFit WODs

For your fitness entertainment, I have compiled 21 individual CrossFit training sessions – aka WODs (or *workout of the day*). Each one will present a unique physical challenge while providing a fitness focus. And, depending on how you approach them, you could have inadvertently stumbled on a veritable goldmine of exercise ideas.

For example, you could complete one of the WODs each day and circulate through them until you've had your fill. Alternatively, you could focus on one WOD a week and look to achieve your best possible time. This approach will provide you with months of training sessions and some healthy competition.

But before you pit yourself against the sessions, it might be worth familiarising yourself with CrossFit terminology. This way you'll know your AMRAPs from your EMOMs and your WODs from your RFTs. Also, by acquainting yourself with the lingo, you'll be able to dive straight into each session without having to pester Google for a definition.

AMRAP

AMRAP is an abbreviation for the training methodology of completing *As Many Repetitions As Possible* in a prespecified time. The process is as follows:

After participating in a whole-body cardiovascular-based warm-up, you would select an exercise, set a countdown timer, and away you go how many reps you achieve nobody knows! That, in a nutshell, is how you would organise and complete an AMRAP.

This training methodology is widely used throughout the CrossFit fraternity for the simple fact that, when it comes to competition, nothing separates the wheat from the chaff like a 20-minute AMRAP.

Furthermore, as a means of advancing physicality – especially in the domains of muscular endurance and strength – the AMRAP is a method par excellence. The ethos is dogmatically centred on volume and max effort. Thus, when you embark on an AMRAP – whether it be 5, 10, 15 or 20-minutes in duration – your primary objective should always be one of striving to achieve the highest number of repetitions physically possible.

EMOM

EMOM is an abbreviation for the training methodology of completing a specific number of exercise repetitions *Every Minute On the Minute*. Though it is a very simple form of training, deceptively so, it is popular among CrossFitters for two reasons.

First, because it is fiercely time-constrained, EMOM brings some serious military-style discipline to a training session. When setting that timer – to count either up or down – it's like having a drill sergeant in the room. And woe betide the weakling who fails to initiate the next set at the start of each new minute.

Second, EMOM massively improves training efficiency (so long as you stick to timings of course). Why? After you've completed your set number of repetitions, say 10 barbell thrusters, there is usually only just enough time on the clock to recover before the minute elapses thus triggering the next set. During an EMOM session there's no time to update your social media account or flirt with your reflection.

WOD

The *Workout of the Day* (or WOD – in case you missed it) is a training session prescribed by CrossFit affiliate gyms and offered to their members. These sessions are disseminated daily – hence the name – to provide members with a training focus and inspire competition. It is cultural convention of the CrossFit fraternity for trainers to 'post' their workout scores on some species of social media. Allegedly this is a means of motivating other CrossFitters to push beyond their perceived physical limitations and not, as some have maintained, to inflate already oversized egos. But that's a barbell of contention for fans to snatch over.

Typically, a WOD can be completed (by an elite level athlete) in under 20-minutes – so about 30-minutes for us mere mortals. However, don't let that put you off. CrossFit workouts, so sayeth the website, 'can be modified to help each athlete achieve their goals' and the 'workouts may be adapted for people at any age and level of fitness.'

RFT

Rounds For Time usually consists of a string of exercises. For example: 20 pull-ups followed by 30 push-ups followed by 40 sit-ups followed by 50 squats. The string constitutes one round. For each RFT a specific number of rounds will be stipulated. It is then the CrossFitter's task to complete all rounds in the shortest time possible. RFT training – as with AMRAPs – is a great way to measure performance progression as they can be employed in a similar fashion to that of a fitness test.

A word on the exercises

If you meet an exercise that you have not yet performed, I recommend practicing the exercise to perfection prior to undertaking the training session. Some of the exercises – such as the snatch, muscle-up, and thruster – are complex movements that, certainly to the inexperienced trainer, pose a significant injury risk. Therefore, approach with caution!

Alternatively, if you do come across an exercise that currently resides outside your sphere of ability, substitute it for one that you can perform competently. By way of example, if you have yet to master the barbell snatch, which is a technically challenging Olympic lift, employ the safer single-arm dumbbell snatch instead.

Okay, now you are clued-up on CrossFit colloquialisms, it's time to meet the girls!

Angie	Barbara	Chelsea
For time, complete all reps of each exercise before moving to the next. • 100 Pull-ups • 100 Push-ups • 100 Sit-ups • 100 Squats	RFT: 5 rounds: • 20 Pull-ups • 30 Push-ups • 40 Sit-ups • 50 Squats Rest for three minutes between each round.	30-minute EMOM. Each of the three exercises to be performed in succession on minute every minute. • 5 Pull-ups • 10 Push-ups • 15 Squats
Cindy	**Diane**	**Elizabeth**
As many rounds as possible in 20-mins. • **5 Pull-ups** • **10 Push-ups** • **15 Squats**	**RFT: 21-15-9 reps.** • **Deadlift (80/90% maximal lift)** • **Handstand push-ups**	**RFT: 21-15-9 reps.** • **Clean (60/80% maximal lift)** • **Ring Dips**
Fran	Grace	Helen
RFT: 21-15-9 reps. • Thruster (40/80% maximal lift) • Pull-ups	30 reps for time. • Clean and Jerk (60/80% maximal lift)	RFT: 3 rounds. • 400-metre run • 21 Kettlebell swings (1.5-pood (24kg)) • 12 Pull-ups
Isabel	**Jackie**	**Karen**
30 reps for time. • **Snatch (40/80% maximal lift)**	**For time.** • **1000-metre row** • **50 Thruster (80/90% maximal lift)** • **30 Pull-ups**	**For time.** • **Wall-ball 150 shots (5-10kg medicine ball)**

Linda	Mary	Nancy
(Aka '3 bars of death') Rep rounds for time: 10/9/8/7/6/5/4/3/2/1. • Deadlift (1 to 1.5 X body weight) • Bench press (1 X body weight) • Clean (3/4 body weight)	RFT: ss many rounds as possible in 20-min • 5 Handstand push-ups • 10 Pistol squats • 15 Pull-ups	RFT: 5 rounds • 400-metre run • 15 Overhead squat (40/60% maximal lift)
Annie	**Eva**	**Kelly**
RFT: 50-40-30-20 and 10 reps. • **Double-unders** • **Sit-ups**	**RFT: 5 rounds.** • **Run 800-metres** • **30 Kettlebell swings (2-pood (32kg)** • **30 Pull-ups**	**RFT: 5 rounds.** • **Run 400-metres** • **30 box jumps (24-inch box)** • **30 Wall ball shots (10kg ball)**
Lynne	**Nicole**	**Amanda**
5 rounds for max reps. There is no time component to this WOD. • Bench press (1 X body weight) • Pull-ups	As many rounds as possible in 20-minutes (note number of pull-ups completed for each round). • Run 400-metres • Max rep pull-ups (without stopping or dropping off the bar – kipping is permitted)	RFT: 9, 7 and 5 reps. • Muscle-ups • Snatches (40/60% maximal lift)

General advice

- To reiterate the warning above, some of the exercises are complex and require formative technical tuition. However, don't let that scare you off. Either get lessons, teach yourself (which with patience and perseverance you could achieve a respectable level of lifting competency) or substitute the exercise for one similar that you can confidently perform.
- Use the grid above like a CrossFit WOD to-do list. Tick off each workout and aim to complete all WODs within a specific period of time.

Workout 24
Compound Exercise Pyramid

How it works

This full-body compound workout is organised into a repetition pyramid. The objective is to progress up the repetition pyramid, starting at one rep, until you have completed 10 reps on each exercise.

To clarify, you are not completing one up to 10 reps on each of the compound exercises separately. Begin at the first exercise, deadlifts, perform one repetition then advance to the second exercise, hang clean, and again perform one rep. The workout has been organised this way to facilitate transition fluidity through the exercises. The objective is to complete the pyramids without resting.

When you have progressed through the four compound exercises, go back to the start but this time complete two repetitions. Proceed in this manner until you have reached 10. If you manage to complete all 10 sets (1, 2, 3, 4, 5, 6, 7, 8, 9, and 10!) on each of the four exercises, you will have performed 220 repetitions total.

Key points

- Before undertaking this workout ensure to warm-up thoroughly beforehand. Spend at least 10-minutes engaged in cardio and light lifting. Every couple of minutes increase the intensity a notch or two so that when you finish the warm-up, you're at around 80% of max effort.
- Organise your bar and weights prior to ascending the pyramid. Remember, the higher you go, the harder it gets. So, at some point, it's likely that you'll need to reduce your bar weight.

- Use the grids provided to track and monitor your progress as you climb the repetition pyramids.

Warm-up

- 10-minutes cardiovascular exercise. It's preferable to select a cardio exercise that works all the major muscle groups such as rowing or the cross-trainer.
- After the cardio phase work through a progressive repetition pyramid of the exercises below. Select a light weight and complete just one repetition of each exercise. Concluding the final rep, go back to the first exercise and now complete two reps. Proceed up the pyramid five times in total.

Workout

Deadlift

- Standing in front of an Olympic bar, adopt a shoulder-width stance.
- Bend down and grasp the bar, palms facing toward you. Remember, bend at the knees ensuring to keep the back straight.
- Before lifting take the strain and then, under control, execute a deadlift by standing up.
- As you stand up push the hips forward.
- At the top position, you should be perfectly erect, not leaning back.
- Keeping correct postural form return the bar to the start position. Or, if you're using bumper plates, drop the bar from the top position.

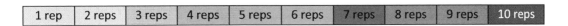

| 1 rep | 2 reps | 3 reps | 4 reps | 5 reps | 6 reps | 7 reps | 8 reps | 9 reps | 10 reps |

Hang clean

- The hang clean start position is the end position of the deadlift.
- So, standing with your feet spaced shoulder-width, hands positioned evenly across the bar and on the outside of your legs, initiate the movement by hinging forward at the hips.

- Using lower back, trapezius, shoulder, and arm strength, pull (clean) the bar up to the front rack position. Throughout its ascent the bar remains close to your torso.
- To assist the initial phase of the movement you can drive the bar up with the hips.
- As the bar is about to sink into the front rack position, rotate the hands ensuring to raise the elbows as you do so. This will ensure that the bar is locked securely in position.
- To conclude the movement, allow the bar to drop into the start position. But it's better to use bumper plates so that you can just release it.

1 rep	2 reps	3 reps	4 reps	5 reps	6 reps	7 reps	8 reps	9 reps	10 reps

Front squat

- The easiest way to get the bar into position to start the front squat is to execute a hang clean. Of course, you'll only be able to do this if you are not going heavy.
- With your feet spaced slightly over shoulder-width, bar supported securely across the anterior deltoids, elbows pointing forward, squat down to 90-degrees.
- When squatting maintain strict form: back remains straight, bending at the knees, no hinging at the hips, and eyes fixed forward.
- At 90-degrees pause momentarily before concluding the movement.
- To conclude the front squat fire evenly through both quads and stand up. Remember, do not lockout at the knees in the top position.

1 rep	2 reps	3 reps	4 reps	5 reps	6 reps	7 reps	8 reps	9 reps	10 reps

Push press

- Following from the front squat, you should already be in the correct position to initiate the push press.
- Your feet are shoulder-width apart, knees slightly bent, supporting the bar under your chin.
- Eyes remain fixed on an indefinite point to your front.

- Taking a shallow dip at the knees, fire through the quads to get the bar moving. This phase of the exercise serves to 'assist' the shoulders.
- Simultaneously engage the shoulders and push the bar above your head.
- Prior to lockout, pause momentarily before returning to the start position for the next repetition.

1 rep	2 reps	3 reps	4 reps	5 reps	6 reps	7 reps	8 reps	9 reps	10 reps

General advice

- In truth, this workout resides in a 'component of fitness' grey area. By that I mean, it's not exactly strength training, neither is it exactly muscular endurance training. It's some weird, mutated merger of the two. Thus, to get through this workout requires the amalgamation and utilisation of both strength *and* muscular endurance.
- Also, because of the point above, knowing how heavy to go, or not to go, presents a dilemma. I suggest starting heavy while you're at the foot of the pyramid, then decreasing the load as you make your climb.

Workout 25
Strength & Fitness Conditioning

What does conditioning mean?

Simply put, *strength and conditioning training* refers to an exercise approach that places emphasis on developing strength, muscular endurance and physical fitness. To engage in strength and conditioning training you need to design workouts that incorporate elements from the main components of fitness.

How do you improve fitness conditioning?

The primary components of fitness conditioning are strength, muscular endurance, cardio and flexibility. If you want to improve your conditioning you will have to focus on developing whole-body fitness. The most effective way to achieve this is by training the main components of fitness in equal measures.

As well as combining cardio and resistance training in your conditioning workouts, you will also have to make room for technique development and flexibility exercises. Remember, conditioning is about enhancing *complete* fitness while also pursuing mastery over exercise techniques.

What are good conditioning exercises?

To improve all-round fitness conditioning, you should organise your workouts so that they include resistance, body weight, and cardiovascular exercises. In addition, you should participate in at least two conditioning workouts per week.

Use the exercises in the list below to create your own conditioning workouts. Do not worry about being formulaic. Pick a handful of exercises arbitrarily, assign distances, reps, and sets, and go for it!

Conditioning Exercises		
Cardiovascular	**Resistance**	**Body Weight**
1. Rowing	1. Kettlebell swings	1. Press-ups
2. Running	2. Kettlebell goblet	2. Triceps dips
3. Cross-trainer	squats	3. Pull-ups
4. Cycling	3. Kettlebell snatches	4. Plank
5. Skipping	4. Dumbbell snatches	5. Air squats
	5. Dumbbell thrusters	6. Burpees
	6. Dumbbell clean to	7. Box jumps
	press	8. Squat thrusts
	7. Farmer's walk	9. Jump jacks
	8. Barbell bent-over rows	10. Hill climbers
	9. Barbell squats	11. Lunges
	10. Barbell military press	12. Step-ups
	11. Barbell hang cleans	
	12. Barbell thrusters	

How they work

The four conditioning workouts below include a diverse mix of exercises and components of fitness. Each workout has been designed around a theme. As well as giving the workouts structure, the themes also improve training focus. When you're armed with a precise training plan, it enables you to get into the zone which minimises procrastination while maximising performance.

You will notice that the four workouts begin with a cardiovascular exercise. This constitutes the warm-up and thus should not be skipped. Concluding the cardio warm-up, progress through the workout following the prescribed exercise ordering.

Key points

- Ensure to complete the cardio warm-up.
- Progress through the list of exercises. Do not deviate from the order.
- There's no need to rush these workouts. You dictate the training intensity.
- However, following from the previous point, if you wanted to compete against the clock, there's nothing stopping you.

Workout 1: Kettlebell and body weight

- 2000-metres rowing
- 5 x 10 reps Kettlebell swings
- 5 x 10 reps plyometrics box jumps
- 5 x 10 reps kettlebell pulls
- 5 x 10 reps press-ups
- 5 x 10 reps kettlebell thrusters
- 5 x 5 reps pull-ups
- 5-mile run (steady pace)

Workout 2: Cardio and calisthenics pyramid

- 10-minutes skipping (or 2000-metres cross-trainer)
- 10 down to 1 press-ups
- 1000m row
- 10 down to 1 box jumps
- 1000m row
- 10 down to 1 air squats
- 1000m row
- 10 down to 1 plank (count the reps as seconds)
- 1000m row

Workout #3: Barbell and resistance band

- 1000-metre rowing
- 5 x 250m row intervals (60% of max effort)

- 5 x 100m row intervals (80% of max effort)
- 3 x 10 reps deadlifts
- 3 x 15 reps resistance band press-ups
- 3 x 10 reps bent-over rows
- 3 x 15 reps resistance band upright rows
- 3 x 10 reps barbell hang cleans
- 3 x 15 reps resistance band lateral raises
- 3 x 10 reps front squats
- 3 x 15 reps resistance band wood chops
- 3 x 10 reps standing shoulder press

Workout #4: Dumbbell into barbell deadlifts
- 5000-metres rowing
- 5 x 15 reps dumbbell squats
- 2 x 10 reps barbell deadlifts (60% of max effort)
- 5 x 15 reps dumbbell bent-over rows
- 2 x 8 reps barbell deadlifts (70% of max effort)
- 5 x 15 reps dumbbell step-ups
- 2 x 6 reps barbell deadlifts (80% of max effort)
- 5 x 15 reps dumbbell lateral raises
- 2 x 4 reps barbell deadlifts (90% of max effort)
- 5 x 15 reps dumbbell thrusters
- 2 x 2 reps barbell deadlifts (100% of max effort)

General advice
- Unless you're blessed with the memory retention prowess of the Rain Man, it's advisable to make a copy of the workouts so you've got something to follow when you get to the gym.
- Organise the training equipment before embarking on the workout.

Workout 26
Smash it for 7-Minutes

First, is a 7-minute workout long enough to promote physiological adaptations? The answer to that question hinges on the intensity at which we train. Studies have shown that even short, high-intensity bursts of between 20- to 30-seconds can promote fat-loss and physical development. And the number of bursts needed to trigger these desirable outcomes is surprisingly low.

For example, in the BBC documentary *The Truth About*, researchers showed that a mere six sets of 20-second high-intensity cardiovascular intervals were enough to burn fat and maintain fitness levels. What's more, after the short duration bursts, the body continued to consume fat for upwards of 20-minutes. Moreover, brief exposures of high-intensity cardio exercise were shown to be effective at stirring a slumbering metabolism.

The 7-minute workout below shares many similarities to those that featured in the aforementioned study. Thus, though surprisingly compact, it still retains the requisite qualities we expect from a training session: that of facilitating fat loss and sustaining fitness levels. An additional attribute of this workout is that you can complete it pretty much anywhere as it requires no equipment. Also, if time permits, you could increase the workout duration by doubling the number of rounds.

How it works

It's advisable to spend a minimum of 5-minutes warming up prior to starting the workout. Once you are sufficiently prepared, set a minute repeater on your training timer and then attack the seven exercises at maximum intensity. There's no stopping for rest, water, or insta pics. Seriously, you've got to assault this 7-minute workout with indomitable determination. And if, after completing the final exercise, you're not wreathing in agony and rolling around in a pool of self-pity, well then you simply didn't train hard enough.

Key points

- *Warm-up!* Remember, warming up improves performance while also reducing injury risk. A double bonus! I know you're sick of hearing me wax lyrical about the importance of warming up, but emphasis enough cannot be heaped on this principle of training.
- I said this workout requires no equipment. That was a barefaced lie. You do need a countdown timer.
- Once warm, and with countdown timer set, smash it for 7-minutes!

Warm-up

- 5/10-minute cardio and calisthenics (jogging on the spot interspersed with squats, burpees, and press-ups – 2 to 5 reps)

Workout

1-minute high-knee raises: simply jogging on the spot while ensuring to raise the knees high so that a 90-degree angle forms at the hip flexor. Deceptively easy, high-knee raises are anything but. I give you 20-seconds before your quads are on fire and you feel like you're going to cough up a lung.

1-minute burpees: a classic military-style exercise that promotes whole-body physicality. When performing burpees ensure that from the crouched position the feet are jumped out and back together. Also, conclude each rep with a plyometric jump. The higher you jump the harder the exercise becomes.

1-minute press-ups: probably the best upper body exercise conceived by mortal man. For this workout try and touch your chest on the floor with each rep.

1-minute plank: gotta love the plank! So simple yet so effective – and as an abdominal toner it has no rivals. Make sure when planking that your back is as straight as, well, a plank. And don't hold your breath!

1-minute hillclimbers: again, another classic military-style exercise that engages a wide range of muscle groups including, of course, the heart and lungs. Though simple, this exercise is often performed incorrectly. Remaining in the high plank (aka the start of a press-up), jump both feet forwards. The knees should brush the outside of the arms before returning to the outstretched position.

1-minute walkouts: a great upper-body and core-strength developer, to perform a walkout you merely walk the hands back from the press-up position until you reach the tip of your toes (or as near as possible). From here, which should see you in the 'downward dog' pose, walk the hands out again until you're back in the press-up position. This exercise can be made an order of magnitude harder by walking the feet up a wall into handstand.

1-minute bastods: the bastod, if you didn't know, is an amalgamation of the burpee and the press-up. From standing drop down into a crouched position, shoot the legs out, perform a press-up, jump the legs back in, stand up and conclude the exercise with an explosive tuck jump.

General advice

- Because you will be working at maximal intensity, it is important to warm-up thoroughly first.
- For performance measures and competition purposes, make a note of the number of reps you achieved for each minute.
- After you've recovered from the physical melee, enjoy a well-earned 5-minute walk or complete the warm-up at a lower intensity.

Workout 27
20-Minute Kettlebell Circuit

This kettlebell workout is a complete training session. In just 20-minutes every major muscle group including a whole host of synergist and stabilisers will be stimulated. In addition, thanks to the functional exercises that feature throughout this 20-minute kettlebell workout, the cardiovascular system is also engaged.

As well as developing functional, multi-muscle strength this short workout will promote fat loss and full-body fitness. The kettlebell deadlift and single-arm press will develop upper body strength in your back and shoulders. In addition to getting the pulse rate up, the kettlebell swing and thruster will improve posterior chain strength and muscular endurance.

Finally, the kettlebell under the leg pass is an effective core-conditioning and coordination-enhancing exercise. According to Pavel Tsatsouline, author of *The Russian Kettlebell Challenge*, 'This drill – a favourite of the Russian military – unexpectedly works the midsection' while also strengthening grip and quad strength.

How it works
First, you are going to warm-up with 10-minutes of either rowing or skipping. After a good warm-up set a 5-minute countdown timer and begin working through the five exercises below.

The objective here is to treat the kettlebell exercises as a mini circular circuit. Start at the first exercise, kettlebell swing, complete 10 repetitions, then move on. Attempt to cycle through the five exercises as many times as you can in 5-minutes.

When the timer sounds finish off the exercise and take a minute rest. Repeat three more times. It's worth marking off every completed lap of the circuit. This way, with each circuit, you'll be able to compete against yourself and tabulate the number of total repetitions performed.

Key points

- Complete a 10-minute progressive warm-up. To improve performance consider throwing in a couple of light rounds of the kettlebell exercise circuit.
- After setting a 5-minute countdown timer, attempt to complete as many cycles of the circuit as your physicality will permit.
- Make a note of every completed lap so that you can convert it into training volume: how many reps you successfully performed in 5-minutes.
- Also, and this just came to me, using your tally chart, you could attempt to exceed your previous number of cycles with each new circuit. Gotta love a bit of self-competition!

Warm-up

- 10-minutes rowing or skipping.
- To better prepare yourself for the workout it is wise, every minute or two, to complete one lap of the circuit. You don't have to complete 10 reps on each exercise, two or three will do.
- Including resistance exercises into your warm-up improves neuromuscular facilitation which better prepares the muscles for the demands of the workout.

Workout

1: Kettlebell swing – 10 reps

- Standing upright grasping the kettlebell between your legs.
- Your palms should be facing inwards, feet a little over shoulder-width apart.

- Maintaining correct posture – back straight, knees slightly bent – pull the kettlebell under your legs and, using glute strength, propel it forward.
- When the kettlebell is level with your shoulder, let gravity return it to the start position.
- Receive the kettlebell with your hips and, using the energy generated, initiate the next repetition.

2: Kettlebell thruster – 10 reps
- Standing over the kettlebell, take a reverse grip of the handle.
- In one smooth movement swing the bell up in front of your chest.
- The kettlebell should be upturned with the base facing the ceiling and your elbows locked at right angles.
- Keeping your back straight squat until there is a 90-degree angle at the knee – or until your forearms touch the top of your quads.
- Fire through both quads powering out of the squat ensuring, as you do so, to push the kettlebell high above your head.
- From the outstretched position lower the kettlebell back to your chest while simultaneously sinking into the next squat.

3: Kettlebell single arm press (jerk) – 10 reps (5 each arm)
- Standing over the kettlebell with a shoulder-width stance (or slightly wider), grasp it and, in one fluid movement, swing it back between your legs and execute a clean.
- The kettlebell should be resting in the nook of your arm and your arm resting on your torso.
- Taking a short sharp dip at the knee, use your quadriceps to get a bit of momentum in the kettlebell. Assist the upward flight with shoulder and arm strength.
- From here, using as little energy as possible, allow the kettlebell to fall back into the nook of the arm. Bend the knees to absorb the impact.
- Immediately initiate the next repetition.
- Complete 5 reps on one arm before changing sides.

4: Under the leg pass – 10 reps

- Stand directly above the kettlebell with your feet spaced a little over shoulder-width. Take the bell from the floor with one hand.
- Keeping your back straight and knees bent, begin threading – or passing – the kettlebell through and around your legs.
- Now trace out a figure of 8 ensuring to maintain a smooth continuous movement for 10 full cycles.

5: Kettlebell deadlift – 10 reps

- Feet firmly planted and spaced about shoulder-width, hold the kettlebell in front of your thighs with your palms facing inwards.
- Hinging at the hips and keeping your hamstrings straight, scrape the kettlebell down your inner calves.
- Engage your core and bring your chest parallel with the floor before standing up.

General advice

- If you've not quite yet got the fitness to attack this workout with the tenacity of a CrossFit athlete, just take your time. There's no shame in that.
- But (following on from above) if you've resolved to go like hell, I advise that you keep track of your circuit cycles so that, when you pluck up the courage to have another crack at it, you'll have a benchmark to compete against.
- Before tackling this feisty little number make sure you are competent on all the exercises. Of course, if you spot an exercise that might cause you a few technical troubles, replace it.

Workout 28
Kettlebell & Body Weight Pyramids

This kettlebell workout is not for the faint of heart. Pitched at an advanced level, for 45-minutes you will have to sustain a high-intensity output if you stand any chance of completing it in the allotted time.

However, if you're up for a tough physical challenge, you've come to the right place. The kettlebell exercises selected for this workout require an experienced level of technical mastery. But don't worry if you think you need to brush up on your techniques, all the exercises are accompanied with a list of key teaching points.

Because this kettlebell workout is supposed to present a challenge you should select a weighty bell. When I had a bash at this one, I oscillated between a 28kg and 32kg kettlebell. By using two different weighted bells you have the option of pushing yourself that bit harder.

Also, for certain kettlebell exercises, such as the swing and squat, you need a heavier bell to feel the exercise working.

How it works
Before embarking on this arduous ordeal, you should warm-up thoroughly. A warm-up organised around skipping and resistance exercises has been provided below. If you are not a competent skipper, select an alternative cardio replacement.

Once warm, start at the first exercise, kettlebell swings, and progress up then back down the repetition pyramid. On completing of each set, you are to perform the same number of repetitions on the accompanying body weight exercise.

To facilitate comprehension of what has been a discombobulating explanation, a diagram has been produced.

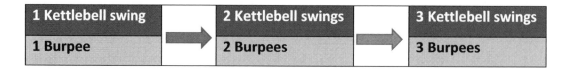

1 Kettlebell swing	2 Kettlebell swings	3 Kettlebell swings
1 Burpee	2 Burpees	3 Burpees

As you can see, the number of kettlebell reps increases in tandem with the body weight reps. The pyramid for all kettlebell and body weight exercises does not exceed 10 repetitions. Emphasis must be heaped on the fact that you are climbing up and then down each pyramid pairing. Example: 1, 2, 3, 4, 5, 6, 7, 8, 9, 10 – halfway, now descend – 10, 9, 8, 7, 6, 5, 4, 3, 2, 1.

Key points

- Oscillating between a kettlebell and body weight exercise, you are progressing up – and then *down!* – a repetition pyramid. So that's one up to 10, then 10 again before you make your descent to where you started – one rep.
- Each pyramid begins with a kettlebell exercise and concludes with a body weight exercise.
- In total, each exercise pairing ascent and descent equates to 220 repetitions. Multiplied by four, if you complete this workout, you'll have performed 880 reps!
- Use the accompanying grids to chronicle your progression and, more importantly, keep track of your position on the pyramid.
- Don't skip the warm-up.

Warm-up

- 10-minutes skipping at varied intensities.
- After every minute stop skipping and complete 10 reps kettlebell swings and air squats.

Workout

1: Kettlebell swings + burpees

- Hold the kettlebell between your legs, palms facing inwards, feet a little over shoulder-width apart.
- Keeping the back straight pull the kettlebell back and, using your glutes, propel the kettlebell forward until it's level with your shoulders.
- Ensuring to keep your core engaged throughout the movement, allow the kettlebell to return to the start position and repeat.

Kettlebell	1	2	3	4	5	6	7	8	9	10
Burpee	1	2	3	4	5	6	7	8	9	10

2: Kettlebell thruster + press-ups

- Standing over the kettlebell, take a reverse grip of the handle – your thumbs point to the body of the bell. In one smooth movement upturn the kettlebell and hold it directly in front of your chest.
- In this position, the base of the kettlebell should be facing the ceiling and your arms locked into right angles.
- Keeping your back straight, squat until your knees are in a 90-degree angle.
- Power out of the squat ensuring, as you do so, to push the kettlebell high above your head.
- From the outstretched position lower the kettlebell back to your chest while simultaneously sinking into the next squat.

Kettlebell	1	2	3	4	5	6	7	8	9	10
Press-ups	1	2	3	4	5	6	7	8	9	10

3: Kettlebell single-arm pulls + air squats

Remember, for the two single-arm kettlebell exercises, you must complete the set on each arm before tackling the body weight exercise. Also, ensure to do all the reps on one arm before changing.

- Place the kettlebell below your centre of mass – you should be standing directly over it.
- Keeping the back straight, squat down, grasp the bell, and stand back up again. The bell should be swinging majestically between your legs.
- Taking a dip at the knee swing the kettlebell back and thrust it forward with the muscles of the posterior chain – hamstrings, glutes, erector spinae.
- Now, this exercise is probably sounding very much like a kettlebell swing. However, the difference is that you pull the kettlebell up to your chin. The kettlebell should remain close to your body similarly to a barbell upright row.

Kettlebell	1	2	3	4	5	6	7	8	9	10
Air squats	1	2	3	4	5	6	7	8	9	10

4: Kettlebell single-arm jerk + plank

There's a slight change with how to approach the body weight exercise. Of course, planks are counted in seconds, not reps. So, instead of performing one rep, as you will do for the previous three body weight exercises, you are to substitute reps for seconds: 1 rep = 1-second, 5 reps = 5-seconds. I think you get the idea.

- Centre you mass over the kettlebell adopting a shoulder-width stance (or slightly wider). Grasp the bell and, in one fluid movement, swing it back between your legs and execute a clean. In this position, the kettlebell should be resting in the nook of your arm.
- Taking a shallow dip at the knee use your quadriceps to get a bit of momentum in the kettlebell. Assist the upward flight of the kettlebell with shoulder and arm strength.
- From here return the bell back to the original start position but ensure to change hands between the legs so that you can perform the next repetition on the opposite side.

Kettlebell	1	2	3	4	5	6	7	8	9	10
Plank	1	2	3	4	5	6	7	8	9	10

General advice

- Print off or make a copy of the exercise trackers so that you can monitor progress. Of course, you can always take the book to the gym and use the trackers I've created for you. I won't be offended if you put ink to this paper – or sweat on it!
- Before attempting this workout, ensure that you can perform all the exercises properly. Poor technique increases injury risk, thus must be avoided like the bubonic plague. If you encounter a kettlebell exercise that you are less than 100% confident at performing, simply swop it for something else.

Workout 29
Go Hercules!

How it works

This workout is dedicated purely to strength development. Thus, between sets, it is advisable to take a substantial rest of 2- to 3-minutes. Long rest periods are important during strength training as the muscles are provided with adequate time to recover for the next lift. By doing so you will be able to shift more weight – which in turn facilitates greater strength gains.

For this strength workout, sets are paired with a prespecified percentage of an assumed maximal lift. So, the first set, you will notice in the table below, features a higher rep range but a lower percentage of maximal lift when compared to those proceeding sets. As the sets progress, reps decrease while percentages increase. Example:

Set number	Rep range	% of max lift
Set 1	10 reps	50%
Set 2	8 reps	60%
Set 3	6 reps	70%
Set 4	4 reps	80%
Set 5	2 reps	90/100%

Remember, the percentage of maximal lift pertains to your personal performance measures – and not to an abstraction from a textbook. Consequently, this workout will yield the best results if you possess an understanding of your current one-rep max (1RM). For without that information, you cannot calculate the prescribed percentages above.

Final point, the only aspect of this strength workout that changes is the exercises. The formula remains the same.

Key points

- Warm-up well before you *Go Hercules!*
- You are focusing purely on developing strength. So, ensure to enforce substantial rest periods between sets.
- Technique is always important when lifting. But arguably it's more so when the weights get heavier. With that in mind, double down on your form and rigidly observe correct lifting procedure: back straight, do not lockout weight-bearing joints, eyes fixed forward, and don't forget to breathe.

Warm-up

- Spend a solid 10-minutes warming up your entire body. I recommend 10-minutes of rowing or pushing and pulling on the cross-trainer. These cardio exercises warm the major muscle groups while also replicating the types of movements that feature in the workout.
- Also, as part of the warm-up, perform one or two light technique lifts of each strength exercise prior to completing the sets.

Workout

Deadlift

- Stand in front of an Olympic barbell or, better still, *inside* a hex bar. (The hex bar, a hexagonal steel structure, is specifically designed for deadlifting. Google it.)
- Assuming that you're using an Olympic bar, grasp it by bending at the knees — NOT rounding at the back.
- Ensure to take the strain *before* lifting and do not 'snatch' the bar off the floor.
- Firing through the quadriceps, stand up ensuring to drive forward with the hips. At the uppermost position, do not lean back. Just stand up nice and erect.
- Return the bar under control.

Bent-over row
- The start of the bent-over row is the top position of the deadlift.
- Hinging at the hips, keeping the back straight, lower down until the bar is level with the top of the knees.
- Eyes fixed forward, row the bar until it touches your stomach – somewhere between your navel and nips.
- Lower under control.

Hang cleans
- Again, as with the deadlift, the start of the hang clean is the top position of the deadlift.
- To initiate the movement hinge forward slightly at the hips and using lower back, arm, and trapezius strength, clean the bar up to the shoulders.
- The top position of the hang clean sees you at the start of the front squat: the bar 'racked' across the anterior deltoids.
- If you're using bumper plates drop the bar. If not, recover under control.

Front squat
- So, in the top position of the hang clean, the bar securely supported in the front rack, space your feet slightly over shoulder-width.
- Keeping the back straight, eyes fixed forward, squat until a 90-degree angle forms at the knee joint.
- Pause momentarily then stand up out of the squat.
- Do not lock the legs in the top position.

Push press
- The bar is in the front rack position. Knees slightly bent. Eyes fixed forward.
- Taking a shallow dip at the knees, use quadriceps strength to get the bar moving.
- Assist with the shoulders as the bar passes the chin – or thereabouts – and press the bar above your head.
- Just before the elbows lockout, pause momentarily.
- Using muscle contraction return the bar to the start position.

General advice

- To ensure that you get adequate rest between sets, consider setting a 2- or 3-minute countdown timer.
- If you plan to attempt a 1RM for the final set, it is advisable to solicit the services of a spotter. It is dangerous to attempt maximal lifts on certain exercises – such as squats and the push press – without support. Ideally, all lifts should be performed on an Olympic barbell clad in bumper plates. This way you can drop the bar if your strength deserts you.
- Calculate the percentages of your current 1RM for the exercises before undertaking the workout.

Workout 30
High-Intensity Interval Training

What is high-intensity interval training?

At its essence, high-intensity interval training (henceforward HIIT) is where we exercise at super-high intensities for short exposures. Typically, each high-intensity interval is immediately followed by a rest or active recovery exercise of equal duration.

The duration of each separate interval rarely exceeds 30-seconds. The reason why is because HIIT training is anaerobic and thus powered by the adenosine triphosphate system (ATP).

Because it's high-octane stuff, and limited in quantity, our stock of ATP is quickly exhausted. Once used up, which at maximal effort takes between 10- to 30-seconds, the body begins synthesising more. However, this takes time.

This is why rest (or active recovery) is an integral component of HIIT training. The rest period between intervals provides the body with enough time to replenish the depleted stock of ATP. Right in time for the next high-intensity interval!

Is HIIT good training?

Yes, most emphatically. HIIT is an excellent exercise methodology for promoting muscular explosivity and superior anaerobic and aerobic fitness.

HIIT sessions, because of the high-intensity element, typically involve cardio and light resistance exercises. Heavy loads aren't completely off the HIIT menu, but the heavier the lift the riskier it becomes – especially so if your technique isn't polished to perfection.

Another attribute of HIIT is that it enables you to pack a lot of exercise into a short space of time. Within a 20- or even 10-minute HIIT session you could comfortably cover more distance or shift more poundage than you could in a 'typical' gym workout (reps, rest, repeat).

And don't be thinking that short duration sessions are in any way inferior to their lengthy counterparts. Recent studies have shown that exercising at high intensities, for as little as 7-minutes, can promote physiological adaptations.

Can anyone train HIIT?

No, not everyone can or should participate in HIIT sessions. Why? If you have a pre-existing injury, even a mild one – such as a muscle strain – high-intensity training could exacerbate the injured area.

HIIT is also unsuitable for untrained people, the elderly, or those carrying excess body fat.

Of course, high-intensity aerobic exercise places significant demands on the cardiovascular system. It goes without saying that this poses a serious risk factor in those who have a weak heart or atherosclerosis – fatty plaque deposits (or 'furring') around the arterial wall.

However, that's not to say that you should never incorporate HIIT into your exercise regime. If you fall into one (or more) of the categories identified above, first work on your general fitness while normalising your body composition – that is, improving the ratio between fat mass and fat-free mass.

When you've improved your cardiovascular fitness and you're at a healthier weight, have a go at a short MIIT session (*moderate*-intensity interval training).

As your fitness develops, you'll be able to change that 'M' to a 'H' and gradually get more adventurous by pitting yourself against the HIIT workouts to follow.

The dos and don'ts of HIIT

Do ensure to participate in a progressive warm-up prior to HIIT. This is arguably the most important aspect of any HIIT session. By progressively warming up the initial interval won't be such a shock to the system. (Think how taxing it is to sprint for a bus from rest – you're bonked before the first 10 steps!)

Also, the warmer you are the better you will perform. The correlation between the two is well established, hence the reason why all professional athletes pay special attention to pre-training warm-ups.

Finally, warming up well can significantly reduce injury risk. (For more on the importance of warming up, and a comprehensive outline of the warm-up protocol, revisit the introduction.)

Don't HIIT with heavy loads, at least not until you have achieved a high level of technical proficiency. HIITing heavy poses a significant risk for beginners and intermediate trainers. This largely results from sacrificing form for intensity. And though we should always maintain flawless form, if we don't the risk factor is not as great if the resistance is low.

Do balance high-intensity intervals with periods of rest and/or low intensity active recovery. The ratio of rest to interval is typically 1:1 – that is, the rest period is equal in duration to each interval exposure. And it is the interval length that determines the rest time.

In saying that, though, you can pretty much do as you please here. However, do bear in mind that, if you take too much or too little rest, it could adversely impact your HIIT performance. This is certainly the case if your rest periods are shorter than the intervals.

Thinking back to the ATP energy system, which once depleted takes time to replenish, if we do not give the body adequate recovery time, our stock of ATP will not have been restored. Thus, we will enter the next interval with an energy deficit.

Don't be afraid to mix cardio and resistance exercises in the same session. There's absolutely nothing wrong with shaking things up a bit by mixing modalities. For example, concluding an explosive cardio row interval you could, after your rest recovery, hit a set of burpees, box jumps, or kettlebell swings. In short, go nuts, experiment, have some fun.

Workouts

HIIT Workout 1: 22 x 300m row sprints
How it works: Your objective is to complete all 22, 300m rows in less than 1-minute each. To achieve this time, you will need to sustain an average pace of 1:40/500. You are to take no more than 1-minute rest between each interval and for the final five sets you are only allowed 30-seconds rest. Make no bones about it, this is a tough HIIT session that transgresses some of the advice above. However, if you feel as though you're not quite physically ready to tackle the session in its entirety, you can modify it by reducing the interval row distances.

HIIT Workout 2: 20-minute skipping and kettlebell swinging combo
How it works: For 20-minutes you are to oscillate between skipping and kettlebell swings. Set a repeating 20-second countdown timer and try to skip as fast and as hard as you possibly can. When the buzzer sounds take your rest. Ensure that you're ready to start swinging the moment the buzzer initiates the next interval.

HIIT Workout 3: 20-minute sprint to air squat
How it works: Applying a similar format as above, for 20-minutes you are to oscillate between sprints and air squats. Set a repeating 20-second countdown timer and try to cover as many metres as you possibly can (it's a good practice to make a note of the number of metres you achieved as this can be used as competition for the next

interval). When the buzzer sounds take your rest. Ensure that you're ready to start air squatting the moment the buzzer initiates the next interval.

HIIT Workout 4: 10-minute calisthenic circuit
How it works: For 10-minutes you are to progress through the circuit below. Set a repeating 10-second countdown timer and try to perform as many repetitions on each exercise station as you possibly can. You will no doubt notice that one full cycle through the circuit takes approximately 60-seconds.

After 10-minutes you will have completed 10 laps. Structuring a session in this way makes it easier to keep track of progression. Also, it's eminently adaptable and if you felt you had enough ATP in the tank, you could go for another five (or 10!) laps.

1: 10-seconds Burpees
10-seconds rest
2: 10-seconds Press-ups
10-seconds rest
3: 10-seconds Mountain climbers
10-seconds rest
Repeat

HIIT Workout 5: 20-minutes boxing to medicine ball slams
How it works: For 20-minutes you are to transition between punching a boxing bag and power slamming a medicine ball – both brilliant exercises and unparalleled fitness developers. So, set a repeating 20-second countdown timer and continuously hit that punch bag as hard as physically possible for the full duration of the interval.

I guarantee that inside the first 10-seconds you'll have spaghetti arms, and your punches will resemble those of a Saturday night drunkard swashbuckling with a streetlamp. When the buzzer sounds take your well-deserved rest. Ensure that you're ready to start slamming that medicine ball the moment the buzzer initiates the next interval.

General advice

- Complete a progressive 10-minute warm-up prior to participating in the preceding HIIT workouts.
- Create a HIIT tracker – or to-do list – and use it to track progress. Ticking off intervals can act as a powerful motivational force.
- Consider recruiting a partner and completing the HIIT workouts together. You can either form a friendship and encourage each other through the intervals or, better by far, regard each other as mortal enemies and compete for physical fame and glory. If you plan on implementing the second suggestion, it works best if you establish punishments/rewards for losers/winners.

Well Done
That's 30 Completed Workouts
Keep Going!

Though the kettlebell is a bewilderingly diverse training tool – boasting more than 25 different exercises – classical Girevoy Sports competitions consist of only three main lifts (or 'events'). These events include the 10-minute snatch, jerk, and long cycle.

Because the jerk and long cycle require twin bells, this workout has been modified to accommodate trainers with one. But, if you have access to two kettlebells, and you can competently perform the jerk and long cycle, then I implore you to go classical.

If you only have one kettlebell, don't think that you're getting off the hook here. For sure, handling two KBs is certainly harder (and not just for the obvious reason that you're lifting double the weight, but more so because it requires significantly more skill to control two bells simultaneously). However, believe you me, one KB will still present a worthy physical challenge.

Kettlebell AMRAPs

Classic kettlebell competitions are comprised of the three events which are organised around the snatch, jerk, and long cycle. The lifter – or *girevik* – has 10-minutes to perform as many quality repetitions as possible. However, there are rules.

Once the 10-minute timer begins, competitors cannot put their kettlebells down. If they are forced to 'down their bells', because of fatigue or a poorly executed lift, they are disqualified from the event.

For a repetition to be counted by the judges, lifters must complete the full range of movement. Any half reps or incomplete exercises and the rep will not feature on the scoreboard.

During the 10-minute snatch, a single kettlebell exercise, the competitor is entitled only to one hand change. Typically, the girevik will start on their dominant arm and snatch for as long as possible before changing. However, over time this leads to strength imbalances and breeds excessive one-sided dominance. To avoid this, the snatch and long cycle will be completed in alternate arm cycles – that is, the hand will change on completion of a short series of reps.

How it works
Split into three individual AMRAPs, your objective is to amass as many repetitions as possible on each of the featured exercises. There are two AMRAP duration options: 5-minutes for beginners and intermediate trainers, and the full 10-minutes for those with an advanced level of fitness.

Unlike the strict Girevoy Sports competitions, the rules outlined above are not enforced. So, if you need to rest your kettlebell during the AMRAP, do so. The moment you feel that you are ready to accrue more reps, pick up your bell and start lifting.

You'll notice that below the kettlebell exercises is a tracker in which you can document your rep scores. The trackers feature three boxes per AMRAP. The idea here, after setting an initial benchmark, is to attempt to beat your previous rep total with each successive attempt. Of course, this works best if you separate attempts with a week or two of intensive kettlebell training.

To recapitulate, your aim here is to amass as many 'quality' reps as possible in the allotted time. This is the only rule that you should enforce. While you are trying to maintain a high output, it is imperative that you observe correct lifting techniques. As the saying goes, quality over quantity.

Key points

- Complete the warm-up.
- Select the AMRAP duration – 5- or 10-minutes – set a countdown timer and see how many repetitions you can amass before the buzzer sounds.
- Take a 2-minute 30-second rest between exercises.

Warm-up

- 2000-metre row, cross-trainer, or skipping at a low- to moderate-intensity. Intersperse the distance with 10-reps of each kettlebell exercise.

Workout

The single-arm snatch

1. Standing over – **NOT** behind! – the kettlebell, adopt a shoulder-width stance.
2. Grasp the bell and, ensuring your weight is on your heels, heave it back between your legs. Your arm should pull into your groin.
3. In one smooth movement drive the bell forward from the hips. You are using the strong muscles of the glutes, lower back, and transverse abdominus to get the bell moving.
4. As the bell sails serenely through the air, assist and guide its flight with your arm.
5. The kettlebell should come to a gentle halt directly above your head.

Note: the kettlebell should swivel around your wrist into position. It must not be allowed to 'flop' over the hand. You'll know if you're applying incorrect technique because after the AMRAP you'll be left with a nasty bruise on the back of your wrist.

5-Minute AMRAP	1st attempt: ……..	2nd attempt: ……..	3rd attempt: ……..
10-Minute AMRAP	1st attempt: ……..	2nd attempt: ……..	3rd attempt: ……..

The jerk (the following technique points apply to single and double bell jerking)

1. To get the kettlebell into position, you'll need to execute a clean: hoist the bell into the nook of the elbow. The folded arm that is cradling the KB should be resting on the upper torso.
2. Once in position and before initiating the movement, organise your feet so that you make a solid base or platform from which to lift. A good solid base will make all the difference when jerking.
3. First, take a shallow dip at the knee and then fire through the quads. To initiate the movement, we use the strong muscle of the quads and glutes – not the shoulder!
4. As the kettlebell begins its vertical trajectory, we help it on its way with a push of the arm.
5. When the kettlebell has cleared the head dip a second time at the knee. Here you are effectively dropping underneath the bell locking the arm out as you do so.
6. At this point the kettlebell should be stationary, your arm straight and knees partially bent.
7. Now stand up.
8. Congratulations! You have completed the first phase of the jerk.
9. To conclude the jerk, simply return the bell back to the nook of the arm and repeat.

Note: as the bell falls into the fold of your arm, you should dip at the knee to absorb the shock of the impact; it also helps to exhale sharply. If you are completing the jerk with a single kettlebell, complete five reps on one arm before changing. Of course, if you change arms after every rep, you'll be performing alternate arm clean and press.

5-Minute AMRAP	1st attempt:	2nd attempt:	3rd attempt: ....
10-Minute AMRAP	1st attempt:	2nd attempt:	3rd attempt: ....

Long cycle (or alternate arm clean and jerk cycle)

1. Stand over the kettlebells adopting a one and half shoulder-width stance.
2. Grasp your bells and, in one fluid movement, swing them back between your legs and execute a clean.
3. In this position, the kettlebells should be resting in the nook of your arm.
4. Taking a shallow dip at the knee, use your quadriceps to get a bit of momentum in the bells.
5. **Don't forget to double-dip!**
6. The first dip, outlined above, initiates the movement. The second dip occurs as the bells pass your head – or thereabouts. Instead of using muscle strength to press the bells above your head, which will hasten fatigue, you are dropping under the bells, locking the arms out, then standing up.
7. Once in the topmost position, pause momentarily.
8. Allowing gravity to do most of the work, retrace your steps in one movement back to technique point three.

Note: there are two natural pause points throughout the long cycle. The first when the bells are nestled in the nook of your arms. The second when pressed overhead. From the overhead position, you do not pause again until the bells are back in the nook of the arms.

5-Minute AMRAP	1st attempt:	2nd attempt:	3rd attempt: ....
10-Minute AMRAP	1st attempt:	2nd attempt:	3rd attempt: ....

General advice

- Master each movement before having a crack at the competitions. Consider spending a week working on your form and then, when you can control the kettlebell like a Russian, pit yourself against the AMRAPs.

- Warm-up well before starting the countdown timer. Also, ensure to incorporate the above kettlebell movements in your warm-up. Just a couple of light sets should do it.
- If you want to imbue your workout with the gloss of Girevoy Sports competitions, solicit the services of a stony-faced second to keep track of your rep score. Oh, and also double the duration of each AMRAP.

Workout 32
3 Measly Minutes

According to some contemporary health professionals, 30-minutes of moderate to high-intensity physical exercise is optimal for improving health and sustaining well-being. (In conjunction with, of course, clean dietary practices, the active avoidance of sedentarism, the abstention of vice (drugs, smoking, alcohol consumption, etc., etc.) and engaging in positive social interactions. There's a bit more to health than meets the eye). This recalibration of the recommended exercise dose is quite controversial.

After all, governmental health advisors encourage the inclusion of 150-minutes of light to moderate-intensity exercise a week. However, few recognise that this duration is merely an 'absolute minimum dosage' that, in truth, is marginally better than doing nothing. If people were told the truth – to wit you should be engaging in some form of exercise EVERY DAY! – most would throw in the towel out of protest at what is to them an unobtainable expectation.

But if you think about it, 150-minutes of weekly exercise is obviously not enough, not when there are over 10,080-minutes in a week. It doesn't take the brains of a NASA scientist to figure out that exercising for (about) 1.5% of the week will not offset sitting on your arse for the remaining 98.5% – or 9,930-minutes.

> I advise one daily "serving" of exercise, which can be split up over the day. I recommend ninety minutes of moderate-intensity activity, such as brisk (four miles per hour) walking or forty minutes of vigorous activity (such as jogging or active sports) every day.
>
> Dr Michael Greger – *How Not To Die* – p. 274

We intuitively know that 150-minutes of exercise across the week is inadequate. Especially when (according to government health advisors) household chores, deadheading your marigolds, and copulating can all constitute 'active' minutes.

More and more health professionals are openly advocating – or prescribing – a minimum daily dosage of 30-minutes. As part of a healthy lifestyle, we should participate in one daily workout consisting of a mixture of cardio, calisthenics, and resistance exercises. The intensity should traverse the spectrum from light to moderate through to high.

To help you implement a daily exercise regime, I have designed an all-purpose whole-body 30-minute workout. Comprised of 10 X 3-minute individual AMRAPs, this workout will stimulate every aspect of your physicality.

Thanks to its innovative design the following workout is fully customisable. Thus, every exercise can be interchanged, and it can be completed in a commercial gym, at home or in your local park.

How it works

On completion of a 10-minute progressive warm-up, you are to work through the following 10 X 3-minute AMRAPs. In 3-minutes you are to perform as many repetitions, or cover as many metres, of the 10 exercises as possible.

Key points

- Warm-up well!
- Set a countdown timer and for three measly minutes you are to sustain a moderate- to high-intensity work rate.
- Progress through the 10 exercises in the order shown.
- Next to each exercise make a note of the number of repetitions and metres achieved. These performance measures can be used to monitor physical improvement or serve as self-competition.
- Take a 1-minute 30-second rest between exercises.

Warm-up

10-minutes cardio and calisthenics.

Workout

1) 3-minutes skipping

Skipping is perhaps one of the best whole-body fitness developers – which accounts for why it is a staple of the boxer's training diet. Bruce Lee said 10-minutes of skipping was as beneficial as a 30-minute run. By that logic, this 3-minute AMRAP is the equivalent of 9-minutes of running – that's some bang for your buck right there! The objective here is super-simple: jump that rope as many times as possible.

2) 3-minutes hanging leg raises

HLRs are more than merely an abdominal toner. They develop core stability and grip strength. In addition, they are eminently modifiable – meaning you can either settle for easy knee raises or test yourself with toes to bar. And if HLRs ever get too easy, which they never do, there's always the option of increasing the resistance by gripping a medicine ball between your knees.

3) 3-minutes cycling

As well as being a Class A cardio conditioner, cycling builds superior stamina while also burning fat like the stuff's going out of fashion. The objective here is to try and cover as many metres as you can in the allotted time. First, set a medium resistance, and then fight tooth and nail to maintain 100-RPM until your run out of road.

4) 3-minutes plank

The plank is a classic core stability exercise. But planking also builds strength in the chest and shoulders. No surprise there considering that you're isometrically holding a partial press-up. If, when imitating a two-by-four, you are required to rest at any point, lest you snap in the middle, pop your knees down, shake the arms out, take a deep breath, and resume the position. The seconds constitute reps.

5) 3-mintes punching bag

Boxing is an immense fitness developer. It enhances cardio fitness, muscular endurance, explosive power … need I go on? Okay then, you asked for it: coordination, agility, speed, reaction time, and, in addition to this panoply of physical attributes, boxing is a brilliant fat burner and muscle toner to boot! Furthermore, as well as training every conceivable component of fitness, you'll also marginally develop your pugilistic prowess.

For 3-minutes you are to throw as many 1-2 combinations as you can – that's a lead left followed immediately by a straight right (reverse if you box out of a southpaw stance). Each 1-2 counts as one repetition and between each combo there should be a distinct but infinitely brief pause: *1-2! … 1-2! … 1-2! …* you get the idea. (But what if I don't have access to a punching bag or pair of gloves? Everything is the same except you are to shadowbox while holding a pair of light dumbbells.)

6) 3-minutes press-ups

I'll be the first to admit that it's somewhat sadomasochistic to position press-ups after punches. For this session planning misdemeanour, no apology will be advanced. Just man up and get on with it. Set a countdown timer, adopt the press-up position, and pump those arms like a pair of well-oiled pistons. How many reps can you rack up in 3-minutes?

7) 3-minutes ergo row

No session is complete without rowing. It's such an awesome exercise and it's enjoyable – at least I think so. The objective here is as unambiguous as objectives get: cover as many metres as your physicality will permit in the specified time. It is recommendable to determine a pace before disembarking. Hold the pace for as long as possible then, for the final 30-seconds, sprint as though your eternal soul depends on it.

8) 3-minutes kettlebell swing

Granted, at this point your forearms should be aflame and your fingers as fragile as warm Kit Kats. Swinging a recalcitrant, gravity-addicted lump of pig iron in such a state is tantamount to torture. But, as the saying goes, what doesn't kill you makes you stronger. Taking the bell off the floor by executing a near-perfect sumo squat, initiate the movement by pulling the bell back into your groin then, firing the glutes, thrust forward propelling it level with your chin. Repeat for 3-minutes.

9) 3-minutes burpees

This exercise that needs no introduction. Just ensure that, when performing this simple yet supremely effective exercise, your feet from the crouched position go out together and, from the press-up position, come back together. Also, don't forget the plyometric jump at the top.

10) 3-minutes run (at 15% incline)

True, running is as old as the hills and is the ultimate no-thrills exercise – which probably explains why it's the least liked (I've never met anyone who enjoyed running). However, few exercises promote cardiovascular fitness and burn fat like quickly putting one foot in front of the other does. And with the added intensity of the incline, you'll forge cast-iron mental toughness too!

General advice

- As with all such sessions, where you are competing against the clock for reps/metres, it's good practice to make a note of your scores. This will provide you with a benchmark to compete against at a later date.
- Though the exercise duration is short, a mere 3-minutes, this workout is still very physically demanding. This is a consequence of the high intensity output you are expected to maintain. However, if you feel that 3-minutes is a bit much for you at present, reduce to 2- or 1-minute exposures. Alternatively, bring the intensity down a notch or two.

Workout 33
10-Minute *HIIT!*

HIIT (high-Intensity Interval) training is a great way to cram a lot of exercise into a short space of time. This 10-minute HIIT workout is the equivalent of an hour-long gym sesh. For 10-minutes you will be exercising at maximum (or near maximum) intensity. Your heart rate will be through the roof, and you'll be fully immersed in maintaining maximal output. During this spicy session there's no time for social media updates or conversations with other trainers. It's all *work, work, work*!

Though it's not everyone's cup of tea, HIIT is a highly focused fitness methodology that enables you to maximise every second of your session. I'm just generalising here but the majority of people who use public gyms spend most of their workout in a state of inactivity. That sounds contradictory I know but if you observe the average gym-goer, you'll see that they waste an awful lot of training time.

One reason for this is that few people follow structured training sessions. Going to the gym without a plan or routine will likely lead to a loss of training focus. However, with this 10-minute HIIT workout, you will have a structured session to follow. And, if at the end of this 10-minute workout you feel like you could do more, you can complete another round or two.

How it works
After completing the warm-up, you are going to work through the four exercises below. On your training timer set a 20-second countdown followed by 10-seconds. For 20-seconds you are to attack the exercise with everything you've got. Once the buzzer sounds take your well-earned 10-second rest. Repeat this format for 2-

minutes 30-seconds. In total, you should complete five high intensity sets for each of the four exercises.

Methods of modification

Don't feel like you've got to follow this 10-minute HIIT workout to the letter. The plan below need only act as a template. You can change any of the exercises to suit your preferences or equipment availability.

For example, if you don't use a public gym, you may not have access to a running machine or rower. But that's not a problem because the run can be performed outside (or you could sprint on the spot), and you could substitute skipping for rowing.

The same goes for the two resistance exercises. If you haven't got access to a kettlebell, you could replace it with a pair of dumbbells or an Olympic barbell and perform thrusters instead. Static double-footed jumps into burpees (taken as one exercise) is just as effective as jumping onto a plyometrics box.

Key points

- Make sure you warm-up well before attempting the HIITs. HIITing when cold is a recipe for injury. Don't put yourself at risk and warm-up.
- Once you've turned the heat up, a lick of sweat glistening across your brow, proceed to attack each interval below.
- Ensure to follow the exercise ordering as per the plan.
- Use the HIIT grids provided to keep track of progress.

Warm-up

- 5/10-minutes progressively warming up on the cross-trainer or rower.
- Throughout the warm-up it would be wise to include resistance exercises structured around ascending repetition pyramids.

Workout

1. Rowing

Rowing is an indomitable fitness developer. And because it activates the two largest muscle groups – those of the legs and back (and the heart!) – rowing provides a brilliant whole-body workout while also stimulating the cardio-respiratory system. These fitness benefits, and there's many more left unmentioned, make rowing a must-have exercise in any training session.

HIIT	REST	HIIT	REST	HIIT	REST	HIIT	REST	HIIT	REST
20	10	20	10	20	10	20	10	20	10

2. Kettlebell swings

So simple yet so effective. Kettlebell swings have been shown to fire up the metabolism like no other exercise. But they also keep the metabolism ticking over for up to 30-minutes after training. In addition, swings are an awesome whole-body strength and muscular endurance developer. And, if you're feeling a bit feisty, you can increase the intensity by putting some extra *oomph!* into the kettlebell propelling it high above your head.

HIIT	REST	HIIT	REST	HIIT	REST	HIIT	REST	HIIT	REST
20	10	20	10	20	10	20	10	20	10

3. Running

Running makes for an excellent HIIT exercise. When that buzzer sounds just do a Captain Kirk and punch it from nought to warp speed. If you're using an indoor treadmill, it's best to keep the belt spinning. Stopping and starting the belt takes yonks. By the time you've got the infernal contraption up to speed, the interval will have finished. So, quick tip, set your desired pace *before* initiating your first HIIT interval.

HIIT	REST	HIIT	REST	HIIT	REST	HIIT	REST	HIIT	REST
20	10	20	10	20	10	20	10	20	10

4. Plyometric box jumps into burpees

Plyo box jump into burpee is a veritable beast of an exercise. A combination of two highly functional calisthenic movements, your entire body, including your cardiovascular system, will receive a ruddy good workout. The movement is initiated with an explosive double-footed jump onto a box (about 2- to 4-foot high). After dropping down the opposite side pop straight into a burpee. Then repeat. The objective here is to maintain a methodical pace. Because of the multifaceted nature of the movement, it's not practical to go fast. But then this exercise is so demanding that you won't need to so long as you keep continuous for the full 20-seconds.

HIIT	REST	HIIT	REST	HIIT	REST	HIIT	REST	HIIT	REST
20	10	20	10	20	10	20	10	20	10

General advice

- Consider making a note of the rep number and distance achieved for each interval. Aim to advance on your previous performance.
- HIIT workouts are ideal for group fitness sessions. See if you can round up a team of sadomasochists and suffer in the company of your comrades.
- Remember, if 10-minutes isn't long enough, double or triple the time. This workout is eminently modifiable and there are a million and one permutations.

Workout 34
A Compendium of CrossFit EMOMs

The following four CrossFit EMOM workouts will help build superior strength. In addition, they can forge functional fitness while also enhancing muscle endurance *and* improving all-round physicality.

The benefits of CrossFit EMOM workouts

In recent years CrossFit has exploded in popularity with affiliated gyms popping up all over the country. But it's no surprise that CrossFit has caught on as well as it has, what with the super-muscled competitors and enviable feats of physical strength.

The slew of YouTube videos and documentaries of hulking athletes battling it out in multi-disciplinary fitness events inspired millions to adopt the CrossFit training methodology. And as people started to discover, CrossFit training can confer loads of fitness benefits.

By dint of design, CrossFit demands that competitors become physical 'Jack of all trades', master at none. In many respects similar to Mixed Martial Arts, which is an amalgamation of all combat sports, CrossFit athletes must ensure that they have no chinks in their armour. It's not enough for a competitor to be strong. They must also develop cardio fitness, muscle endurance, and a whole host of other physical attributes.

Across the four days of CrossFit competitions, athletes are put through a gruelling series of fitness challenges – sometimes up to three separate events each day. The challenges could include anything from Olympic lifting, swimming events, marathon row and strongman complexes.

To prepare for such a diverse range of disciplines, CrossFit athletes must cultivate a high degree of competency in multiple components of fitness. The only way to achieve this, of course, is by incorporating all exercise methodologies and disciplines into their training regime.

If you begin including CrossFit-inspired workouts into your routine, you too may develop complete fitness.

Four CrossFit EMOM Workouts

10-minute EMOM – Thruster Disguster

Whether you love them or loath them (most people harbour the latter feeling), you cannot deny that the barbell thruster is an awesome compound exercise. This single movement will develop supreme quad, core, and deltoid strength.

Furthermore, because barbell thrusters engage such a wide range of muscle groups, they also stimulate the cardiovascular system. Meaning that, in addition to developing whole-body conditioning, thrusters can also build cardiac muscle tissue which will improve the strength of the heart.

- EMOM: 10 X 1-minute barbell thruster (aim for 10 reps for the first 5-minutes and 15 reps for the second 5-minutes)

Total reps: 150

20-minute EMOM – Macho Man

I'll be straight with you, I filched this workout from a CrossFit YouTube video. In the video Matt Fraser, five times CrossFit champion, along with a crew of other dedicated CrossFitters, worked through a clean and press complex.

But instead of performing the exercise in one movement, it was broken down into three parts: power clean, front squat, overhead press. They completed three reps on each of the separate movements, totalling nine reps per minute. This doesn't sound like a lot, I concede. The average time each athlete took to execute the nine reps was 20-seconds, leaving 40-seconds recovery.

However, the movements are complex, which means they must be approached with extra caution, and the weights were high. I think Fraser was throwing around a 90kg barbell.

Depending on your current level of fitness, it might be worth starting this workout with a light bar. As you progress through the rounds, incrementally increase the weight. This approach will improve your chances of completing the entire workout without compromising form.

- EMOM 20 X 1-minute: 3 reps deadlifts, 3 reps hang cleans, 3 reps overhead press – 9 reps total.

Total reps: 180

30-minute EMOM – Raw Power

Following a similar theme from the preceding workout, for 30-minutes you will progress through a clean and press complex.

Again, the exercise is broken into its three constituent parts: deadlift, front squat, and push press. But where this workout differs from the one above is that each exercise forms its own EMOM workout.

So, the first EMOM sees you perform 12 deadlifts on the minute every minute for 10 rounds. The following two 10-minute EMOM workouts are the same except that the exercises change.

For the advanced trainer, or those wanting to push themselves, there is an optional challenge. If you've got enough gas in the tank, you can pit yourself against the full clean and press over 5 X 1-minute rounds. The reps are low, a mere six, but it's a horrid exercise.

- EMOM 1: 10 X 1-minute deadlifts (aim for 12 reps)
- EMOM 2: 10 X 1-minute front squats (aim for 12 reps)
- EMOM 3: 10 X 1-minute overhead push press (aim for 12 reps)
- EMOM 4: 5 X 1-minute clean and press (aim for 6 reps)

Total reps: 360 (390 including the challenge)

40-minute EMOM – The Beast

As the saying goes, save the *beast* till last. The final EMOM workout is a compendium of CrossFit exercises. Comprised of a mix of calisthenics, functional movements, and Olympic lifts, this EMOM brings you the full CrossFit experience. But in doing so it will test every aspect of your physicality.

It starts off deceptively easy and thus can lull you into a false sense of security. After the first 10-minutes, you'll think you've got this one in the bag. But the intensity picks up precipitously as you enter the second set of 10-minutes, which starts with a set of dumbbell thrusters into a plyometric burpee. *Oh, the pain!*

From there this EMOM workout gets messy. And with 30-minutes of exercise remaining, if you hope to see the final round you've got to be prepared for a tough physical fight.

- EMOM 1: 10 X 1-minute 4 reps box jumps + 4 toes to bar
- EMOM 2: 10 X 1-minute 6 reps dumbbell thrusters + 4 bar jumps into burpees
- EMOM 3: 10 X 1-minute 6 reps single-arm dumbbell snatch (3 reps each arm) + 4 reps kip pull-ups
- EMOM 4: 10 X 1-minute 4 reps barbell power cleans + 4 reps barbell thrusters

Total reps = 360

General advice

- Some of the exercises that feature throughout the above EMOMs are a touch more technical than those of your typical training sesh. Thus, it's wise to acquaint yourself thoroughly with the technical application of complex exercises before tackling the EMOM.
- If you focus on each workout for a week, you have a whole month of training here.

Workout 35
The Kettlebell Snatch

If you've got limited time to get your fitness fix, or you just want a quick whole-body blast, this kettlebell snatch workout is the ideal training session for you. In a mere 15-minutes this workout hits every major muscle group including your cardiovascular system.

But 15-minutes of kettlebell snatching does more than activate a wide range of muscle groups. The snatch also builds grip and posterior chain strength like no other exercise.

In addition, if you incorporate this short session into your general training regime, you'll also start to develop superior muscular endurance and explosive power.

It begs the question, though, can a single kettlebell exercise deliver all those fitness benefits?

Snatch | Tsar of the kettlebell exercises

In short, yes, the kettlebell snatch is a serious strength-developing exercise that packs an unparalleled fitness punch. But if you don't believe me, here's what Pavel Tsatsouline, author of *The Russian Kettlebell Challenge*, has to say:

'The one-arm snatch is the Tsar of kettlebell lifts, fluid and viscous. It will quickly humble even studly powerlifters. The forces generated by this drill are awesome. "How can it be if the weight is so light?" you might ask. – Through great acceleration and deceleration. Would you rather roll a 500-pound barbell over your toes or drop a 72 pounder from seven feet? I rest my case.'

In addition to the tremendous forces generated when snatching, the exercise transitions through multiple joints. In doing so the snatch activates all the major muscle groups as well as a whole host of smaller synergists and stabilising muscles.

How it works

Organised around ascending pyramids, this workout is broken up into three 5-minute AMRAPs. The objective is to progress as far up the pyramid as possible in the allotted time.

But it's not all about snatching! Between each snatch set, there is a calisthenics exercise that you are to complete before progressing up the pyramid.

The method is as follows. After starting a 5-minute countdown timer, complete one rep snatch on each arm followed by one press-up. (The body weight changes with each new AMRAP.) Now just add another rep to each exercise.

Continue in this fashion until you run out of time. Don't forget to make a note of your scores at the end of each AMRAP as you can use this to compete against next time.

Key points

- You're going to warm-up well so that your muscles will be ready for the snatching onslaught to come.
- After setting a 5-minute countdown timer, proceed to ascend the snatch-to-calisthenics exercise pyramid.
- Remember, your objective is to climb as high up the pyramid as possible in 5-minutes.
- Don't forget that when snatching you must perform an equal number of reps on each arm.
- If you run out of time mid set, ensure to complete it prior to resting.
- Before moving to the next 5-minute AMRAP, treat yourself to a 2-minute 30-second recovery break.

Warm-up

- Suggested 10-minute warm-up: 2000-metre row interspersed with kettlebell swings and light snatches.
- After rowing 250-metres, dismount and complete 5 repetitions of the two kettlebell exercises. Repeat until you've covered 2000-metres.

Workout

5-minute AMRAP: Snatch to press-up

Kettlebell Snatch	1	2	3	4	5	6	7	8	9	10	11	12
Press-up	1	2	3	4	5	6	7	8	9	10	11	12

5-minute AMRAP: Snatch to air squat

Kettlebell Snatch	1	2	3	4	5	6	7	8	9	10	11	12
Air squats	1	2	3	4	5	6	7	8	9	10	11	12

5-minute AMRAP: Snatch to burpee

Kettlebell Snatch	1	2	3	4	5	6	7	8	9	10	11	12
Burpees	1	2	3	4	5	6	7	8	9	10	11	12

How to perform the perfect kettlebell snatch

If you're new to snatching, you should know that there's more to the exercise than meets the eye. From experience, on the rare occasions that I've observed this exercise being performed, incorrect technique is always applied. There are a few technical nuances that typically slip beneath the radar of most snatchers.

However, if the snatch technique is mastered, it makes the exercise far less unpleasant to perform. For example, you'll finish your workout with fewer blisters and sores on the palms of your hand, and you won't be left with a nasty bruise on the back of your wrist. Furthermore, applying correct form also improves movement efficiency which slows the onset of fatigue. To help you get the most out of this 15-minute workout, below you will find a step-by-step snatch tutorial.

But it goes without saying that there's only so much you can learn from a written description. To perfect the snatch technique, you must practice, practice and *practice!*

And finally, if you are new to snatching, ensure to start off with a light kettlebell and focus on the intermediate movements before piecing them together.

Snatch teaching points

1. Centre your mass over a kettlebell ensuring to adopt a stance slightly over shoulder-width.
2. Keeping your back straight squat down and grasp the bell then stand back up again.
3. Initiate the movement by pulling the bell between your legs.
4. Once you feel the bell push you back, your arm taught against your torso, fire through the glutes and core while simultaneously pulling with the back muscles.
5. **Remember:** you are not 'lifting' with your arms, but rather propelling the bell with your hips. The arm merely acts to control and guide the trajectory of the kettlebell.
6. If you've put enough 'umph' into the bell it should sail up smooth and sweet. But you're not swinging it out like you would with a single-arm swing. You must cut the trajectory short and aim to keep the bell close to your body.
7. Before reaching the top position, the bell should swivel round the back of your wrist. This positional transition ought to take place with the mechanical precision of a Swiss watch. Basically, what I'm trying to say is the bell shouldn't 'flop' over the hand slapping against the back of the wrist. But you'll soon know

if you're not doing it right because the following day your wrist will be bruised and sore.

8. To recover the movement, rotate the bell back round the wrist and allow the kettlebell to drop like a pendulum to the start position.

9. Harness the generated energy to initiate the next rep.

Snatching dos and don'ts

✓ Do select a weight commensurate with your current ability.

✓ Do keep that back straight.

✓ Do adopt a stance slightly over shoulder-width: you do not want that bell thwacking into your kneecap as it does the big dipper!

✓ Do hold your unencumbered arm out to aid balance.

⊗ Don't snatch near your ma's finest China.

⊗ Don't allow the bell to pull you down so that your torso becomes parallel with the floor. Performed properly, the snatch is quite a compact movement. The common mistake is to overemphasise the rotation at the hips as the bell bowls through the legs. When performed incorrectly, as has just been described, you'll see a 90-degree angle form at the quads and abdominals. The angle formed at the hips needn't exceed 45-degrees.

⊗ Don't 'swing' the kettlebell out as you would a swing. Instead, after you've propelled it forward with the strong muscles of your glutes and transverse abdominus, pull it up. Comparative to the swing, when snatching the bell should remain relatively close to your body.

Workout 36
Skip and Swing Sesh

This skipping and kettlebell workout burns fat, builds functional strength, and improves whole-body fitness. But then it's no surprise that this workout confers all these benefits, considering it is comprised of arguably two of the best exercises in existence.

Skipping is widely acknowledged as a superlative fat-burning exercise. As well as incinerating fat, skipping also improves muscle definition. By including skipping into your general training routine, it won't be long until you start seeing visibly sharper muscle separation. But regular skipping won't just make your muscles more defined, it also improves endurance and cardiovascular performance.

Whereas skipping takes care of cardio and muscle endurance, the kettlebell exercise will help build strength in the major muscle groups. The kettlebell is a celebrated functional fitness developer, which accounts for why it is so popular among the fitness fraternity.

For this workout, we'll be focusing only on the kettlebell swing. The swing is a powerful foundational exercise that improves posterior chain and core strength. Other fitness benefits associated with kettlebell swinging include gorilla-like grip strength, enhanced muscle endurance, and improved whole-body fitness.

How it works
At its essence, this skipping and kettlebell workout is uber-simple. Your objective is to complete as many skipping and kettlebell swing sets as possible in 10-minutes. To

make this workout accessible to a wider audience, it has been organised into three levels. They are as follows:

- Beginner: 25 skips to 12 kettlebell swings (12/16kg)
- Intermediate: 50 skips to 25 kettlebell swings (16/24kg)
- Advanced: 100 skips to 50 kettlebell swings (24/32kg)

Key points

- Select the level commensurate with your current fitness ability. As your fitness and skipping skills improve advance to the next level.
- As previously stated, the objective of this workout is to complete as many of the above sets as possible in 10-minutes. To achieve the best possible score, you should aim to skip and swing nonstop for the entirety of the workout.
- But of course, you do not have to pursue that objective. Instead, you can take rests between sets if you feel the need.
- If you do decide to rest, I advise sticking to a specific duration – say 10, 20, or 30-seconds – to avoid exercise procrastination. To improve discipline, consider setting a countdown timer.

Warm-up

Before skipping spend 2- to 3-minutes performing mobility exercises. Mobility exercises involve controlled rotations of the joints: ankle rotations, knee bends, high knee raises, etc. Once you're feeling a little more mobile, start double-footed skipping. This will further warm and limber up the gastrocnemius muscles (calves) and Achilles tendons.

I labour the pre-workout warm-up explanation because skipping cold can cause calf and/or Achilles tendon twinges. Jumping straight into a skip session (no pun intended) is an act of folly that could easily result in an injury. Don't fall foul to this training trap.

Workout

Beginner	Intermediate	Advanced
25 skips **12 kettlebell swings** **(12/16kg)**	**50 skips** **25 kettlebell swings** **(16/24kg)**	**100 skips** **50 kettlebell swings** **(24/32kg)**
25 skips 12 kettlebell swings (12/16kg)	50 skips 25 kettlebell swings (16/24kg)	100 skips 50 kettlebell swings (24/32kg)g
25 skips **12 kettlebell swings** **(12/16kg)**	**50 skips** **25 kettlebell swings** **(16/24kg)**	**100 skips** **50 kettlebell swings** **(24/32kg)**
25 skips 12 kettlebell swings (12/16kg)	50 skips 25 kettlebell swings (16/24kg)	100 skips 50 kettlebell swings (24/32kg)
25 skips **12 kettlebell swings** **(12/16kg)**	**50 skips** **25 kettlebell swings** **(16/24kg)**	**100 skips** **50 kettlebell swings** **(24/32kg)**
25 skips 12 kettlebell swings (12/16kg)	50 skips 25 kettlebell swings (16/24kg)	100 skips 50 kettlebell swings (24/32kg)

Make this a 20-minute skipping and kettlebell workout

If 10-minutes is too short for you, or you wanted to make this skipping and kettlebell workout into a full training session, simply double (or triple!) the duration. Of course, if you do opt for 20-minutes, you'll have to temper the intensity at which you work.

By selecting the 20-minute workout you can also incorporate different kettlebell exercises (such as the snatch which, if you completed Workout 35, you should well be a master at). With more training time at our disposal, the workout dynamics are not disrupted as much when transitioning between exercises.

General advice

- To help keep track of the number of skip/swing sets you've completed, consider using the above grid to track your progress.
- If you want to increase the intensity of this workout, there are two ways to achieve this. Way 1: do double-unders for the last 10 skips of each set. Way 2: swing the kettlebell above your head.

Workout 37
EMOM Madness

Each of the EMOM workouts below will bring structure, discipline, and a whole lot of physical fitness to your training regime. But if you're new to the EMOM methodology (or you missed Workout 34 – A Compendium of CrossFit EMOMs) and you've got some questions about this contemporary form of training, turn to Appendix A where you will find a full explanation of the EMOM training methodology.

Key points

- A 'How it works' introduction heads each EMOM workout.
- Complete a 10-minute warm-up before doing battle with the four EMOMs. Instead of producing a proscriptive warm-up, some suggestions have been posited below.
- The warm-up overview is suitable for all the workouts that follow.

Warm-up

- Before completing the four EMOM workouts spend 5- to 10-minutes warming up.
- Best warm-up exercises include whole-body cardiovascular exercises such as rowing, skipping, and the cross-trainer.
- Interlace through your warm-up a series of body weight exercises – press-ups, air squats, and burpees all engage big muscle groups.
- Alternatively, complete a repetition pyramid (1 up to 5) comprised of those exercises that feature in the EMOM.

EMOM Workout 1: Body weight

The first workout is ideal for beginners and those new to EMOM training. Here you will be tackling four 5-minute EMOMs. Each workout focuses on a different body weight exercise. Because there is no additional resistance involved (other than your body weight of course) and the exercises are simple, you should aim for a higher rep target.

Suggested rep targets accompany each exercise. Remember, though, they are only suggestions and thus can be amended and tailored to suit your level of fitness and ability.

5 x 1-minute press-ups (20 to 40 reps)
5 x 1-minute squat jumps (20 to 30 reps)
5 x 1-minute pull-ups (5 to 12 reps)
5 x 1-minute burpees (10 to 25 reps)

EMOM Workout 2: 20-Minute complete conditioning

The objective of this EMOM is to provide you with a whole-body training session. This workout includes resistance, body weight, and cardiovascular exercises. So, while developing muscular strength and endurance, you'll also improve your cardio fitness as well.

5 x 1-minute bastods (10 to 20 reps)
5 x 1-minute rowing (100 to 200-metres)
5 x 1-minute kettlebell swings (10 to 20 reps – 12/16/24/32kg bell)
5 x 1-minute hang cleans into overhead press (6 to 12 reps – 40 to 60% of max lift)

EMOM Workout 3: 30-Minute total strength builder

This workout is organised around the clean and jerk. Instead of completing the exercise in its full form, it has been broken down into its constituent parts. You will spend 6-minutes on each part with the option of piecing the parts back together and going for an additional 6-minutes for the full exercise.

Aim for a target of between 8 to 12 repetitions. Of course, the weight you select will largely determine your rep target. It is good EMOM practice to increase the load when you progress into the latter part of the workout. So, you could, as an idea, aim for 12 lighter weight reps for the first 4-minutes then increase the weight and reduce the reps for the final 2-minutes of each set.

6 x 1-minute deadlifts (8 to 10 reps – 60 to 80% of max lift)
6 x 1-minute hang cleans (8 to 10 reps – 40 to 60% of max lift)
6 x 1-minute front squats (8 to 10 reps – 60 to 80% of max lift)
6 x 1-minute standing shoulder press (8 to 10 reps – 40 to 60% of max lift)
6 x 1-minute complete clean and press (8 to 10 reps – 40 to 60% of max lift)

EMOM Workout 4: 20-Minute kettlebell clean and press
Following the theme above, we're going to split the kettlebell clean and press into two parts each forming its own EMOM. Again, there is the option of increasing the duration and intensity of this workout by piecing the two parts back into one complete movement.

Also, if you're feeling up to the challenge, you can slip a 10-minute kettlebell thruster (or goblet squat) EMOM between the clean and press. By doing so you'd turn this into a monstrous workout.

10 x 1-minute clean (8 reps (4 reps each arm))
10 x 1-minute thruster (8 reps) (optional)
10 x 1-minute press (8 reps (4 reps each arm))
10 x 1-minute clean and press (6 reps (3 reps each arm)) (optional)

General advice
- You don't have to stick to the suggested repetition targets. For example, let's say you're going to work through a 10-minute deadlift EMOM. Initially, you set the rep target at six. Instead of sticking to that target, consider incrementally

increasing the rep count by one repetition every minute. This technique both significantly increases training volume – especially if you're EMOMing for 20-plus-minutes – and intensity.

- It's a self-imposed rule of mine that when I enter the last minute I do not stop until the timer sounds. I set myself the challenge of doubling the standard rep target over the final minute. This is the EMOM equivalent of a sprint finish. Feel free to follow suit.

- Remember, it's not a written rule that you have to stick with the same weight throughout your EMOM workout. It is good training practice to change up gears throughout any workout by either a) increasing reps or b) increasing weight. By adding more weight to your resistance exercises you will force the muscles to work harder which in turn will encourage strength gains. Just remember, if you do decide to increase weight, take small jumps as opposed to large leaps.

Workout 38
Boxing Cardio & Calisthenics Combo

If you want to burn calories, trim up, and get fit in the process, you should start including the occasional boxing cardio workout into your routine.

A boxing cardio workout offers an engaging alternative to standard sweat sessions.

Instead of forcing yourself on that obligatory long slow run (so dull!), you could mix things up a bit by putting yourself through a fat-busting boxing workout.

As well as disintegrating calories and enhancing whole-body fitness, boxing can also help bust stress. And another great thing about boxing workouts is that they require hardly any equipment or space.

But don't you have to be a boxer to train like one?

No! This is a common misconception that's resulted in many people missing out on the benefits of the boxing training methodology. You can enjoy boxing workouts without fighting or throwing a punch at a fellow human being.

To take part in this boxing session all you need is a skipping rope, a bit of space for body weight exercises, and a resistance band. That's it!

Boxing cardio workout benefits

Though this boxing cardio workout won't transform you into the next world champion, it will provide you with a new training dynamic. One that will stimulate your physicality in different ways and hopefully inspire you to include more boxing-inspired workouts into your routine.

In addition to offering some much-needed variation, this boxing cardio workout will put your through your paces. By doing so you'll enjoy a high intensity sweat session that will burn some serious calories.

Boxing workouts build whole-body fitness

Furthermore, because this boxing-inspired sweat session features calisthenics exercises as well as cardio, your whole body will be actively engaged.

Thus, while promoting cardio fitness and consuming a week's worth of calories, this workout improves endurance and muscular tonality.

Boxing training fights fat

Boxing is one of the best training methods for burning fat. The reason why boxing burns calories so effectively is because it is high intensity and involves lots of cardiovascular exercises. Most all boxing sessions start with either a 30-minute run or 20- to 30-minute skip. And that's just part of the warm-up!

Moreover, unlike more traditional training methods (gym-based sessions), boxers take very little rest during a workout. As a consequence, they maximise their training time by eking the most out of each exercise minute.

And because the majority of the workout is spent sweating, as opposed to resting, posing, or switching between exercise equipment, much more energy is expended. If more energy is expended, then more calories are consumed. If more calories are consumed, then there's less to be stored as fat.

Key points
- Below there are three separate workouts: basic, medium, horrible (I mean *hard*). The titles assigned to each workout speak for themselves.
- If you want a moderately relaxed session, perhaps to be used as a pre-session warm-up or post-weightlifting workout pulse raiser, go basic.

- But say you fancy a bit of challenge, maybe that circuits class didn't live up to expectations, or you need to atone for an over-indulgent weekend, medium is for you. It'll put you through your paces but won't leave you feeling (or looking!) like Rocky after going twelve with Apollo Creed.
- For those who want to go toe-to-toe with The Manassa Mauler, there's only one workout for you, and that's horrible (obviously). This is a nasty session that will induce a hellish cardio burn.
- And for those true fitness sadomasochists (or the wannabe Rocky Balboas), dare to do all three workouts – on the bounce!

This boxing cardio workout includes skipping!

To maximise the fitness outcomes of this boxing cardio workout, it's helpful if you can competently skip. That is, maintain a fluid consistent skipping action for minutes at a time while also being able to pop out a burst of double-unders without tying yourself in knots.

The three workouts are primarily structured around skipping and involve 'jump rope' HIIT blasts.

However, if your skipping skills are on par with that of a primary school girl (no offence to primary school girls), you'll be glad to know not all is lost.

You can substitute skipping for short shuttle sprints or jogging on the spot. But skipping is preferable by far.

How to skip like a seasoned pugilist

For those who can skip, but just haven't done so in a while, below you will find a technique refresher.

If you have never skipped, or you were one of those unfortunate people born with two left feet (no offence to people with two left feet), jettison the skipping and settle for sprinting.

Step 1: WARM-UP! Your warm-up should consist of ankle and knee mobility exercises. Also, air squats, light bounces, and low-intensity plyometric jumps should be incorporated into your pre-skipping warm-up.

Step 2: While holding the rope in your hands, practice double-footed jumping – you are not skipping yet, just practicing the mechanics. Spend 1- to 2-minutes doing this.

Step 3: Holding the handles loosely, the rope at rest behind you, turn it over and jump the rope once then stop.

Step 4: Repeat Step 3 for 1- to 2-minutes.

Step 5: Now attempt to jump the rope as many times as possible without stopping. Ensure to count the number of jumps you achieved as you are going to try to beat it next time.

Step 6: For 5-minutes work on sustaining a consistent skipping action.

Warm-up

Before attempting any of the boxing workouts below, ensure to warm up thoroughly first. Ideally, your warm-up should be consistent with the workout and feature similar – preferably the same – exercises.

To make life easy for yourself, you could complete the basic workout at a low intensity. This will suffice as a suitable whole-body warm-up while also providing you with a feel for the session structure.

1: Basic workout

The basic boxing cardio workout is short and sharp making it ideal for a warm-up or to cap a weightlifting session. Remember, if you can't skip shuttle sprint for the same duration.

- 1-minute skipping (aim for 80 revolutions per minute)
- 1-minute shadowing boxing

- 1-minute body weight exercises: 5 burpees - 5 press-ups - 5-seconds plank - 5 squat jumps
- **Rest 1-minute**
- 2-minute skipping (aim for 80 revolutions per minute)
- 1-minute shadowing boxing
- 1-minute body weight exercises: 5 burpees - 5 press-ups - 5-seconds plank - 5 squat jumps
- **Rest 1-minute**
- 3-minute skipping (aim for 80 revolutions per minute)
- 1-minute shadowing boxing
- 1-minute body weight exercises: 5 burpees - 5 press-ups - 5-seconds plank - 5 squat jumps
- **Finish or repeat**

Total workout time: 15-minutes

2: Medium workout

At almost double the duration of the basic, the medium boxing cardio workout would suffice as a session on its own. In addition to the increase in rounds, you are also required to maintain a higher skipping output – 90 revolutions per minute. Also, you'll notice that the skip duration increases with each successive round.

- 2-minute skipping (aim for 90 revolutions per minute)
- 1-minute shadowing boxing
- 1-minute body weight exercises: 5 burpees - 5 press-ups - 5-seconds plank - 5 squat jumps
- **Rest 1-minute**
- 3-minute skipping (aim for 90 revolutions per minute)
- 1-minute shadowing boxing
- 1-minute body weight exercises: 5 burpees - 5 press-ups - 5-seconds plank - 5 squat jumps
- **Rest 1-minute**

- 4-minute skipping (aim for 90 revolutions per minute)
- 1-minute shadowing boxing
- 1-minute body weight exercises: 5 burpees - 5 press-ups - 5-seconds plank - 5 squat jumps
- **Rest 1-minute**
- 5-minute skipping (aim for 90 revolutions per minute)
- 1-minute shadowing boxing
- 1-minute body weight exercises: 5 burpees - 5 press-ups - 5-seconds plank - 5 squat jumps
- **Finish or repeat**

Total workout time: 26-minutes

3: Horrible workout

The final boxing cardio workout is a 45-minute slugfest that will put even the fittest pugilist through their paces. As with the medium, the number of rounds has increased along with the skip duration. But a couple of other intensifiers have been thrown into the fight.

You now must maintain 100 skip revolutions per minute. No mean feat I can tell you, especially when the skip duration increases with each round. Also, you are to change up the gears over the final 20-seconds of each minute by performing double-unders. Ouch! Oh, and keep your eyes peeled for that cheeky 3-minute skip finish before the final bell.

And finally, when shadowboxing you should fasten yourself into a resistance band – of between 20 to 30kg resistance. (If you haven't got access to a resistance band, hold a pair of 3kg dumbbells instead.) This will put a nasty burn in the shoulders and tire the arms out for the body weight exercises.

- 2-minute skipping (aim for 100 revolutions per minute – double-unders last 20-seconds)

- 1-minute shadowing boxing (with a 20kg resistance band or 3kg dumbbells)
- 1-minute body weight exercises: 5 burpees - 5 press-ups - 5-seconds plank - 5 squat jumps
- **Rest 1-minute**
- 3-minute skipping (aim for 100 revolutions per minute)
- 1-minute shadowing boxing (with a 20kg resistance band or 3kg dumbbells)
- 1-minute body weight exercises: 5 burpees - 5 press-ups - 5-seconds plank - 5 squat jumps
- **Rest 1-minute**
- 4-minute skipping (aim for 100 revolutions per minute)
- 1-minute shadowing boxing (with a 20kg resistance band or 3kg dumbbells)
- 1-minute body weight exercises: 5 burpees - 5 press-ups - 5-seconds plank - 5 squat jumps
- **Rest 1-minute**
- 5-minute skipping (aim for 100 revolutions per minute)
- 1-minute shadowing boxing (with a 20kg resistance band or 3kg dumbbells)
- 1-minute body weight exercises: 5 burpees - 5 press-ups - 5-seconds plank - 5 squat jumps
- **Rest 1-minute**
- 5-minute skipping (aim for 100 revolutions per minute)
- 1-minute shadowing boxing (with a 20kg resistance band or 3kg dumbbells)
- 1-minute body weight exercises: 5 burpees - 5 press-ups - 5-seconds plank - 5 squat jumps
- **Rest 1-minute**
- 5-minute skipping (aim for 100 revolutions per minute)
- 1-minute shadowing boxing (with a 20kg resistance band or 3kg dumbbells)
- 1-minute body weight exercises: 5 burpees - 5 press-ups - 5-seconds plank - 5 squat jumps
- 3-minute skipping (aim for 120 revolutions per minute)
- **Finish or repeat**

Total workout time: 45-minutes

General advice

- Before skipping ensure to warm-up well. Begin by spending 2- to 3-minutes performing ankle and knee mobility exercises: controlled rotations, bounces, and light plyometric jumps. Only after the mobility phase should you start jumping rope.
- To maximise your performance and get the most out of this workout, you need to be able to skip competently. Remember, though, all is not lost if you can't skip – you'll be sprinting instead. However, consider putting in some practice on the rope and, when you can sustain a consistent work rate, come back for a rematch.

Workout 39
High-Intensity Interval Skipping

This skipping HIIT workout promises to send your cardio fitness into the stratosphere. As well as being one of the all-time best whole-body exercises, skipping is also a brilliant fat burner and metabolic conditioner.

Martial arts legend and fitness fanatic Bruce Lee purportedly proclaimed that skipping is one of the most effective single exercises we can do. He also apparently claimed that 10-minutes of skipping was as physically demanding as 30-minutes of running.

If Lee is right, and jumping rope is three times more effective than jogging, then this skipping HIIT workout is like going for a 1-hour 15-minute run. Yet you'll only be skipping for 25-minutes.

Skipping HIIT benefits

This skipping HIIT workout will provide you with a challenging training session. One that will leave you feeling like you've pushed yourself to your fitness limits. Also, another benefit of this skipping workout is that it requires only a jump rope and a bit of space. So, you can complete it almost anywhere – at home, on holiday, or at work over a lunch break.

In addition, because the workout is organised into three HIIT series, consisting of one 5-minute and two 10-minute blocks, the duration of the workout can easily be tailored to suit your time constraints. But if you can find a permanent place in your training programme for this skipping workout, you stand to gain other fitness and health benefits besides those already outlined.

More benefits

- ✓ Improved cardio performance
- ✓ Enhanced muscular endurance
- ✓ Fat loss
- ✓ Improved body composition
- ✓ Visibly sharper muscular definition

How it works

Before having a go at this workout ensure to warm-up for 5- to 10-minutes. Begin by spending a couple of minutes completing mobility exercises: ankle rotations, knee bends, high knee raises . . . you know the drill. After the mobility exercises start skipping.

Once warmed and ready to go, set a 10-second repeat timer. Your objective is to work through the three HIIT series below.

Grouped into one 5-minute and two 10-minute blocks, you're skipping at a high intensity for 10-seconds before taking a rest of the same duration. However, each HIIT series gets more challenging as the interval duration increases while the rest remains the same and then decreases.

On conclusion of each high-intensity interval, it's recommendable to tick over at a low intensity for the rest period. Of course, you can stop to rest if you feel the need, but it can make it all the more challenging to get going again.

Key points

- Faithfully follow the pre-workout warm-up protocol.
- You'll be oscillating between interval and rest for a combined total of 25-minutes.
- This workout is comprised of three skipping HIIT series that progressively increase in intensity.
- On completion of each HIIT series, take a 2-minute rest.

Warm-up

- To echo the same warm-up advice proffered in the Skip and Swing Sesh (Workout 36), ensure to spend 2- to 3-minutes performing mobility exercises before you start jumping rope.
- Mobility exercises, remember, involve controlled rotations of the joints: ankle rotations, knee bends, and high knee raises.
- Concluding the mobility exercises, complete about 50 controlled double-footed plyometric jumps.
- You should only start skipping when your calves and Achilles tendons are warm and limber.
- Once you've started skipping proper, progressively raise the intensity.

Workout

First HIIT series

The first HIIT series consists of thirty 10-second interval/rest pairings. Though the interval duration is short, the intensity should be near maximal – meaning 100%, throw-the-kitchen-sink at it.

1-minute	Interval	Rest	Interval	Rest	Interval	Rest
2-minute	Interval	Rest	Interval	Rest	Interval	Rest
3-minute	Interval	Rest	Interval	Rest	Interval	Rest
4-minute	Interval	Rest	Interval	Rest	Interval	Rest
5-minute	Interval	Rest	Interval	Rest	Interval	Rest
6-minute	Interval	Rest	Interval	Rest	Interval	Rest
7-minute	Interval	Rest	Interval	Rest	Interval	Rest
8-minute	Interval	Rest	Interval	Rest	Interval	Rest
9-minute	Interval	Rest	Interval	Rest	Interval	Rest
10-minute	Interval	Rest	Interval	Rest	Interval	Rest

Second HIIT series

Concluding the rest, reset the repeating interval timer but this time for 20-seconds. Following a similar format as outlined above, complete this HIIT series for another 10-minutes. Again, on completion take another 2-minute rest.

1-minute	Interval	Rest	Interval
2-minute	Rest	Interval	Rest
3-minute	Interval	Rest	Interval
4-minute	Rest	Interval	Rest
5-minute	Interval	Rest	Interval
6-minute	Rest	Interval	Rest
7-minute	Interval	Rest	Interval
8-minute	Rest	Interval	Rest
9-minute	Interval	Rest	Interval
10-minute	Rest	Interval	

*Note the back-to-back interval leading up to the final minute.

Third HIIT series

For the final HIIT series, you will be skipping at a high intensity for 20-seconds. But you'll only get a 10-second rest. This minor reduction in rest really cranks up the heat. Getting through the intervals requires more than just fitness: you'll also need grit and determination.

However, whereas the previous two HIIT series are scheduled for 10-minutes, the final challenge is only 5-minutes in duration. Don't let that lure you into a false sense, it's still a beast.

1-minute	Interval	Rest	Interval
2-minute	Rest	Interval	Rest
3-minute	Interval	Rest	Interval
4-minute	Rest	Interval	Rest
5-minute	Interval	Rest	Interval

General advice

- Ensure to warm-up thoroughly before tackling the HIIT workout.
- To help you keep track of progress, consider using the interval grids above. After each interval/rest pairing put a line through the box. It's a bit like bingo except the only prize for a full house is fatigue and sweat . . . and a sense of satisfaction.
- If you can, avoid stopping completely during the rest periods. Try ticking over at a low intensity. Alternatively, you could shadowbox or perform air squats.

Workout 40
4-Week Strongman Training Programme

Something different for you . . .

First, before we consider the how, the following question ought to be answered: *why bother training like a strongman?*

For starters, strongman exercises are typically functional in nature. When executing a barrel lift or tyre flip, say, two staples of the strongman diet, a veritable legion of muscles must work in synchronicity.

Furthermore, because the exercises are compound movements, they transition through multiple joints which improves biomechanical coordination while stimulating muscular adaptations – that is, developing the density and mass of muscles (aka *hypertrophy*).

It is this multi-muscular attribute of strongman exercises that forges functional physicality and raw power. A fitness development duo that delivers superior performance results. These positive outcomes transcend those conferred by conventional gym-based static and isolation lifting.

In addition to augmenting physical robustness, strongman training can also build mental toughness. There's no getting away from the fact, power cleaning kegs, heaving heavy hammers, tossing tractor tyres, and lumping about loadstones (if you happen to possess any), batters and bruises the body. As a consequence of this corporal conditioning, you'll inevitably develop a durable disposition and those once challenging gym sessions will feel like a day out at the spa.

172

More benefits of strongman training

Improved body coordination

Functional exercises, unlike their inferior static counterparts, require that we move across unconventional planes. For example, the classic strongman exercise Farmer's walk, engages the body in ways that singular isolation movements could not. I see static lifting as two dimensional, whereas functional training is three dimensional.

Augmented biomechanical synchronicity

Functional exercises require the deft coordination of multiple body parts while exerting force against a resistance. Thus, by dint of necessity, strongman training develops biomechanical mastery.

Enhanced proprioception

Complex, multi-dimensional movements demand continuous conscious engagement. When performing a series of hammer tyre slams, say, or heaving a heavy dumbbell over your head, you can't lapse into a daydream. Certainly not like you can when seated comfortably on the leg press machine. The inherent complexity of functional training forces a unification of mind and body which brings about a strengthening of neural pathways: aka proprioception.

Re-correcting strength imbalances

The physical strength of the trainer who engages predominantly in static exercises tends to represent a set of scales overladen on one side. Yes, they might boast a 220 bench, or 330 dead, or 440 squat, but when they're required to exert force outside of a two-dimensional plane their true strength shows its meek face. Picture the Adonis who, with bulging biceps and an inflated chest, can scarcely perform a single tyre flip without inducing cardiac arrest.

Functional exercises, on the other hand, which are the hallmark of strongman training, develop the body in unison and strength imbalances are quickly exposed. Two logical outcomes follow from this. First, the trainer gives up and goes back to the gym. Second, the trainer perseveres and in so doing rectifies the imbalances.

Strongman kit is relatively cheap and surprisingly easy to procure

Contrary to popular opinion you don't have to spend a fortune on strongman equipment. For precisely zero pounds I procured a 150kg tyre, 65kg aluminium beer keg (minus the beer), and a sled. How? You may well ask. Simple. While out cycling I spotted a disused tractor tyre in a farmyard. I asked the farmer politely if he mind me adopting it. He didn't. I peddled home furiously, begged my better half to drive me back, and subsequently rolled that recalcitrant ring of rubber two miles to my doorstep. Yeah, I got some unwanted attention, but you can't pass up an opportunity for quality training kit.

The barrel I 'appropriated' from a derelict pub and, as for the sled, I got a friend of mine, a plumber by trade, to weld it together from factory offcuts and half-inch thick cast-iron plates.

As well as being cheap – or, if you're prepared to scavenge, beg, borrow and steal, free – strongman equipment is eminently durable. In a thousand years' time, I'll be little more than scattered dust, but my strongman kit will be as good as new. Especially my sled, that thing's invincible!

Benefits of strength training

Strength is usually pursued as an end in and of itself. Usually, because the strong man (or woman) receives backslaps, adulation, and kudos from fellow gym frequenters and the physically enfeebled. As physical attributes go strength is by far the most coveted. This has been the case for thousands of years. In the Iliad Homer sings the praises of the strong man – the indomitable Ajax and the wrestling feats of Odysseus – and it was Hercules' strength alone that carried his name through the ages. However, when acquired in this mindset – to be strong because it carries considerable social coin – strength is almost worthless. Honestly, in the real world, when's Billy Big Arms ever going to be called up to curl 100kees?

But when used to enhance performance in activities – such as a sporting discipline like swimming or rowing – augmented strength is highly beneficial. In the brilliant book *Physical Fitness & Athletic Performance*, Watson cites a study showing performance gains made by elite-level athletes after adopting a strength training programme. A mere 'four weeks of strength training produced a 19 per cent increase in power which resulted in a 4 per cent improvement in swimming speed.'

Purported benefits of strength training include
- ✓ Increased muscle mass
- ✓ Increased strength
- ✓ Stronger tendon and ligaments
- ✓ Increased metabolic rate
- ✓ Anti-ageing benefits
- ✓ Reduced fat
- ✓ Increased bone density
- ✓ Reduced blood pressure
- ✓ Reduced blood cholesterol and blood fats
- ✓ Improved posture
- ✓ Reduction in injury susceptibility
- ✓ Improved psychological well-being
- ✓ Improved appearance

(List adapted from Anita Bean's *Strength Training: The Complete Guide To*)

Strongman training approach

Now that we've considered the many associative benefits, let's turn our attention to strongman training approaches. However, there's one crucial point to bear in mind before embarking on a strongman-inspired training programme. That is, heavy lifting places greater stress on the joints, muscles, ligaments, and tendons. Thus, if you fail to execute near flawless form and/or train too often, you significantly increase the risk of incurring an injury. To reduce injury susceptibility, ensure always to:

- Thoroughly warm-up before engaging in strongman/strength training
- Progressively increase loads throughout the session

- Master the lifting techniques on lighter loads first
- Ensure to rest for one to two days between strongman sessions
- Employ the support of a training partner if possible
- Provide the body with adequate, quality nutrition post-training (to aid recovery)
- Implement a post-session rehabilitation routine – stretching and foam rolling
- **DO NOT EVER** try to lift more than you are physically capable
- And always value the *quality* of the lift over the *quantity* of the load lifted

To start a strongman training programme, you will of course need access to the appropriate equipment. If you haven't followed in my footsteps, and gone out on the pinch, strongman kit can easily be procured nowadays: you're only ever two clicks away from an Amazon delivery van depositing a tractor tyre on your doorstep. However, if you're too tight-fisted to part with your pennies, most of the exercises that feature in the strongman programme can be simulated with standard gym equipment.

But assuming that you do have access to kegs, tyres, and sleds, below you will find a 4-Week Strongman Training Programme based on that of a professional strongman competitor. For those used to gym training, CrossFit or circuit training, the programme will appear a little parsimonious; that is, it doesn't contain a lot of exercises, reps, and sets. There's a reason for this.

The training protocol for improving strength is to reduce sets and repetitions while increasing loads and rest periods between lifts. Arnold Schwarzenegger said that to develop his impressive size and strength he 'included a lot of heavy' lifting in his routine and, he tells us, when trying to build strength and size, 'you need to train according to basic power principals – fewer reps and sets, more rest between sets, but with increased poundage,' (*The Encyclopaedia Of Modern Bodybuilding* – p.493).

Also, unlike cardiovascular and muscular endurance training, which require considerable volume to make noticeable physical development, significant strength gains can be achieved with surprisingly few sessions.

For example, in her book *Strength Training | The Complete Guide To*, Anita Bean cites research showing 'that a basic weight training programme lasting just 25 minutes, three times a week, can increase muscle mass by about 1kg over an eight-week period, while lean mass gains of 20 per cent of your starting body weight are common after the first year of training.'

So, in summary, when transitioning from a more involved training routine to that of one predicated on strength/strongman principles, it is important to curtail volume and focus more on poundage, lifting technique and, of course, rest, recovery, and nutrition. For as Bean put it, though often overlooked or underestimated, these factors all play a 'crucial part of a strength training programme.'

(**Please note**: the programme is supposed only to serve as a guide and offer a general outline of how a strongman regime could be structured.)

		Hungry4Fitness **4-Week Strongman Training Programme**		
	Week 1	**Week 2**	**Week 3**	**Week 4**
Monday Lower Body	Farmer's walk – 3 X 25m Squats – 3 X 10 reps Sled drags – 3 X 25m	Farmer's walk – 3 X 50m Squats – 3 X 10 reps Sled drags – 3 X 50m	Farmer's walk – 4 X 75m Squats – 3 X 10 reps Sled drags – 3 X 75m	Farmer's walk – 5 X 100m Squats – 3 X 10 reps Sled drags – 3 X 100m
Tuesday	**Rest Day** **Relax, Recover, Replenish**	**Rest Day** **Relax, Recover, Replenish**	**Rest Day** **Relax, Recover, Replenish**	**Rest Day** **Relax, Recover, Replenish**

Wednesday **Hip Extension**	Deadlifts – 3 X 8 reps Hang-cleans – 3 X 8 reps Tyre flips – 10min AMRAP*	Deadlifts – 3 X 8 reps Hang-cleans – 3 X 8 reps Tyre flips – 12min AMRAP	Deadlifts – 4 X 8 reps Hang-cleans – 3 X 8 reps Tyre flips – 14min AMRAP	Deadlifts – 5 X 8 reps Hang-cleans – 3 X 8 reps Tyre flips – 15min AMRAP
Thursday	**Rest Day** **Relax, Recover, Replenish**	**Rest Day** **Relax, Recover, Replenish**	**Rest Day** **Relax, Recover, Replenish**	**Rest Day** **Relax, Recover, Replenish**
Friday **Upper Body**	Military press – 3 X 8 reps Barrel carry – 3 X 25m Kettlebell swing toss – 10min AMRAP	Military press – 3 X 8 reps Barrel carry – 3 X 50m Kettlebell swing toss – 12min AMRAP	Military press – 4 X 8 reps Barrel carry – 3 X 75m Kettlebell swing toss – 14min AMRAP	Military press – 5 X 8 reps Barrel carry – 3 X 100m Kettlebell swing toss – 15min AMRAP
Saturday	1-hour swim/cycle or combination of cardiovascular activities	1-hour swim/cycle or combination of cardiovascular activities	1-hour swim/cycle or combination of cardiovascular activities	1-hour swim/cycle or combination of cardiovascular activities
Sunday	**Rest Day** **Relax, Recover, Replenish**	**Rest Day** **Relax, Recover, Replenish**	**Rest Day** **Relax, Recover, Replenish**	**Rest Day** **Relax, Recover, Replenish**

*AMRAP: as many repetitions as possible

General advice

- *What's a kettlebell swing toss?* Well, since you asked, it's where you explosively swing a kettlebell over your head and toss it as far behind you as possible. I probably needn't posit this caveat but do ensure that you're not in a public place when executing this exercise.

- But you don't have to toss your bell! Instead, execute a full swing sending the kettlebell above your head. This minor adaptation will still confer considerable strength gains.

- It stands to reason that you will encounter an exercise(s) in the programme that, for whatever reason, you are unable to perform. If this possible eventuality manifests into reality, don't sweat it! Simply substitute the exercise for one which possesses comparable characteristics and similarly stimulates the body.

- By way of example, let's say that you don't have a tyre to flip. Listen, that's not the end of the world and other exercises can be recruited to fill the void of that tyre. A terrific whole-body strength developer – which is perhaps in some ways superior to tyre flipping – is car pushing. Yep, you read that right: car pushing. A friend of mine used to perform this exercise all the time – and he was incredibly strong (and incredibly strange). He'd ask the 'missus' (his vernacular) to maintain a steady course and apply the brakes when approaching solid objects while he pushed his car up and down the road. Granted, there are a million and one limitations to this exercise (if it can be called that). But if you live in a quiet cul-de-sac and you care not a crap about your street credibility, then this could just be the perfect replacement for tyre flips. Alternatively, perform deadlifts.

Well Done
That's 40 Completed Workouts
Keep Going!

Workout 41
The Power of Fitness Testing

Unless you test yourself, you stagnate.

Mark Allen – winner of six ironman titles

Before we can improve our fitness, we must first know how fit we are. That sentence is as tautological as they come but how many people do you know who test themselves on a regular basis? Personally, I don't know any.

The conspicuous absence of fitness testing among exercise enthusiasts probably accounts for why so few trainers push themselves beyond their current level. Though this is of no surprise because we only become aware of our fitness levels through testing.

A fitness test provides us with an unbiased insight into our current level of physicality. Depending on the test selected, we can gather detailed, accurate, and near-instant information regarding our strength, muscular endurance, and cardiovascular capacity.

By shedding light on our physical strengths and weaknesses, by exposing the chinks in our fitness armour, so to speak, we are able to begin the process of rectifying imbalances and striving towards augmented physicality.

This can provide us with a goal and an area of focus.

Exercising without these two things – a goal and area of focus – is equivalent to setting sail without a destination. Consequently, most trainers are adrift, floating aimlessly from one unproductive training session to the next.

Fitness testing gives us a starting point. It says *You are here*! How important those three words are cannot be understated. After all, if we do not know where we are, then knowing where we are going and if progress is being made along the way are impossible.

Once we have a start point, we can chart a destination. This provides us with a goal to aim for while also imbuing our training with purpose.

Benefits of fitness testing
✓ It can prevent physical stagnation as we have a goal to work towards
✓ It imbues our training with purpose
✓ Testing can reignite dwindling motivation
✓ It can encourage us to push beyond perceived physical limits
✓ It can bring structure to our training regime
✓ It can expose physical weaknesses that can then be corrected through the modifications of training practices
✓ Provides a means of monitoring training effectiveness and progress

The aim of this workout
The aim of this workout is to provide you with a range of fitness tests to try. In addition, I have outlined the protocol that should be implemented prior to conducting a fitness test. But why bother observing testing protocol?

By adopting a laissze-faire attitude towards testing – say the distance or time is inaccurate, or the conditions under which the test was conducted made it unreproducible – the results become increasingly unreliable.

Unreliable results are almost as unhelpful as no results at all. In fact, they are arguably worse. Inaccurate fitness test data could corrupt our perception of out true physical capability. This undesirable outcome could be avoided (or at least significantly minimised) if we had taken the time to ensure testing consistency. And, if we're going to invest time into testing our fitness, we might as well strive to be as accurate as possible.

Each test comes accompanied (where applicable) by a normative data set. This is important because, if we have no information relating to previous performances of the test, we have no measure against which to compare our attainment. Thus, we are clueless as to whether we've done well or not.

However, in saying that, the normative data can be dismissed, and you can use the tests merely as a means of monitoring personal progression. It is fine to adopt this approach.

So, when conducting the 2000m ergo row test, for example, you could record your time with the view of improving it in a month or two. Perhaps to monitor performance development as part of the marathon row training programme (Workout 50). Using fitness tests independently of normative data is fine when the focus is purely on personal improvement.

Furthermore, due to the glaringly obvious fact that most all recognised fitness tests provide the trainer with an extremely parochial insight into their physicality, you can design your own broader test. Though this comes with the limitation of an absence of normative data (not to mention the near impossibility of maintaining reliability), it will, like the example above, inform you of fitness gains made.

(On that note, many of the circuits and workouts in this book can be used as a means of tracking physical progression. For example, those workouts that encourage you to time your performance, act as a quasi-fitness test.)

Think VRR when fitness testing

Before we take a look at the fitness tests, I shall first outline a number of important factors that should be considered prior to conducting any test. As I mentioned above, if we are careless in our testing the outcome measures – the results – will be inaccurate. Inaccuracies are not only misleading but also invalidate future re-test outcomes.

Thus, when we test, we must do so methodically ensuring to strive for the most accurate outcome. The factors that ought to be considered prior to conducting a fitness test are:

1: Validity
2: Relevance
3: Reliability

Validity

Before undertaking a fitness test, you must ensure that it will provide you with an insight into the desired component of fitness. 'The validity of a test indicates the extent to which a test measures what it sets out to measure,' (Watson 1995). So, before busting a gut over a 1.5-mile run, or inducing cardiac arrest on the 2000m ergo row, you should ask yourself: is this test going to provide me with the fitness measure I am seeking?

However, I may have jumped the gun here. Before we determine if a test adheres to the stipulations imposed by the concept of validity, we need to decide which component of fitness we wish to measure. The components of fitness include:

1: Muscular endurance
2: Muscular strength
3: Cardiovascular
4: Power
5: Speed
6: Flexibility
7: Agility (skill-based measure)
8: Coordination (skill-based measure)
9: Body composition (health measure)

Once you have decided which component of fitness you wish to test, you would then select the appropriate fitness test.

Relevance

The relevancy of a fitness test can only be determined if the information it provides is of benefit. You could ask yourself: how will conducting this test support me in my pursuit of improved physicality? Only you can answer that question.

However, if you are not training for a specific sport or discipline, such as a running event or triathlon competition, but are just interested in gaining an insight into your general fitness, then testing cardiovascular performance is the best place to start. Why?

A purist might criticise any attempt to prioritise in order of importance the components of fitness. And even though they all have their place and serve a particular purpose, I doubt few would or could quibble with the contention that cardiovascular is a more insightful fitness measure than strength or flexibility.

I've arrived at this conclusion because cardiovascular tests provide us with an indication of the relative performance capacity of our heart, vascular and respiratory systems.

Moreover, by pursuing cardiovascular fitness we will engage in activities that are synonymous with good health, reduced body fat, and enhanced longevity. The same cannot be so confidently said for strength training and/or flexibility.

Thus, if you plan to include more testing into your training regime, I advise prioritising cardio tests. Better still, mix and match.

Reliability

Before we conduct a fitness test, we must ask ourselves: is this reproducible? Why should this question not only be asked but answered in the affirmative? For the simple reason that the results from the fitness tests are only of use if they can be compared against future results.

If the test cannot be reproduced – perhaps because of how or when or where it was performed – the results will be invalidated.

Furthermore, an unreliable or unreproducible test will almost certainly provide you with unreliable or unreproducible results. And such results are best off in the bin as they can be misleading.

I'm reminded of an incident a good many years back when I was discussing ergo row performances with an acquaintance – as you do. He goaded me into divulging my current 2000m PB (whenever someone does such a thing it's usually a primer for them either to display their perceived physical superiority, usually by submitting a better time, or as a means of comparison – in this case, it was the former).

My ego got the better of me and I promptly supplied my current 2000m ergo row PB. He almost immediately shattered it by stating that he could sustain a 1:13/500 average over the same distance. I fought back the impulse to laugh hysterically, and not for the fact that his physicality more closely suited that of a pub darts player, but because a 1:13/500 average translates to a sub-5-minute 2000m row. At his best, the multi-Olympic champion and man-mountain Matthew Pinsent could pull 5:45.

I asked this acquaintance of mine if he was quite certain about this phenomenal time. He asserted most emphatically that he could maintain 1:13/500 over 2000-metres. I asked him how he could be so sure. He told me that that's what his rower had recorded. I questioned the accuracy of his rower. He staunchly maintained that his rower was the most accurate and reliable rower in existence.

In the end, I left him to his delusion – and I didn't have the heart to tell him that his rower was obviously faulty.

Testing procedure

My anecdote was supposed to illustrate the importance of ensuring that a fitness test satisfies VRR – that it is *valid*, *relevant*, and *reliable/reproducible*. If it doesn't, we run the risk of wasting our time and deluding ourselves in the process.

Below I have created an eight-step procedure that you can implement prior to engaging in any fitness test. Though it is true that no procedure, irrespective of how robust it is, can completely guarantee absolute testing reliability, it can help minimise inaccuracies.

- **Step 1**: Decide which component of fitness you wish to test.
- **Step 2**: Select the appropriate test (see examples below).
- **Step 3**: Determine when and where you plan to conduct the test. (It is wise to make notes of these details so that you can recreate the conditions come the day of the retest.)
- **Step 4**: If equipment is to be used – such as a running machine, rower, bike – ensure that it is accurately calibrated and that the distance is displayed in the appropriate metric. (I mention this because I once organised a group fitness test on indoor stationary bikes half of which were in miles and half in kilometres. I only realised my mistake partway through the test when there were significant distance discrepancies between the participants – as they say, live and learn!)
- **Step 5**: Ensure that the equipment used will be available come retest.
- **Step 6**: Know your plan of attack prior to attempting the fitness test. By this I mean, what strategy of approach will you use? For example, over the 1.5-mile run, which is a standard military cardiovascular test, I have tried numerous strategies over the years in a bid to better my PB. These strategies include starting slow and building pace over the distance; maintaining a high pace throughout; starting fast, falling below pace to raise it again over the remaining half mile. Once you have decided on a plan of attack, make a note of it and be sure to apply it during the retest.

- **Step 7**: Make notes of your pre-test routine. How long before conducting the test did you eat? How were you feeling on the day? What did you do during the hour prior to the test? What warm-up did you complete?
- **Step 8**: Once you have completed the test, make notes of your performance, and ask yourself: how did it go? Did I perform well? If *Yes* why? If *No* why? could I have worked at a higher intensity? Did anything of note happen that impeded my performance?

The Fitness Tests

Prior to conducting a test, and assuming you have followed VRR as best as you possibly can do, you must consider warming up. A warm-up is of paramount importance irrespective of whether you are taking part in an exercise session or pitting yourself against a test.

Warming up not only improves our physical performance but also reduces our chances of injury. For an outline of how to warm-up effectively, refer to the discussion on training principles in the introduction.

Cardiovascular fitness tests

2000m ergo row test

The 2k ergo row is the be-all and end-all of fitness tests. I say this because rowing recruits the two major muscle groups – legs and back – including most all other muscles in-between. Consequently, to keep so many muscles fuelled, the heart and lungs are required to work overtime.

What constitutes a respectable 2k time? An Olympic rower will comfortably go sub-six minutes (1:30/500) – the world record stands at 5:35 which is an average of 1:23.5/500 (that is, 1-minute 23.5-seconds per 500-metres – which is utterly insane).

However, we must bear in mind that, as in boxing, rowers are divided into weight divisions. Heavyweights will pull the big sub-sixes whereas elite rowers from lighter weight categories aim for under 6:30. For non-elite rowers, a time under or around 8-minutes (2:00/500) is worthy of recognition.

As with any test there are multiple strategic methods of approach. Having tried numerous methods over the years in my bid to go sub 6:30, I have found the four-phase method to be the most effective.

Four-phase 2000m ergo row method
The 2k distance is split into four 500-metre blocks. We initiate the first 500m with five huge pulls bringing the pace at least 15-seconds below the target.

After those five big pulls we gradually 'dial in' to our target pace. By the time we are on pace, the first phase will have concluded.

Between phases two and three we strive to maintain a consistent pace at or close to our target. As we exit the third phase, we will be entering the final 500m.

Over the final 500m – which can be further broken down into two 250-metre segments – we aim to hold the pace until that moment when we initiate the sprint.

Other rowing tests
The following tests range from intermediate distances to full and ultra-marathons. Rows of these lengths are approached quite differently to the 2k erg as explained above. The pace remains consistent and comfortably within the aerobic training zone. Also, considerable preparation is required before tackling such tests (see Workout 50). Opposite the five distances, current best times have been included.

- 5000m (14:56)
- 10,000m (31:05)
- 21,090 (half marathon) (1 hr, 7 min)
- 44,195 (full marathon) (2 hr, 21 min)
- 100,000m (6 hr, 6 min)

1.5-mile military run test

The 1.5-mile run is the cardiovascular test of choice throughout the British military. Though the attainment times vary across the different services, the objective remains the same: cover the distance as quickly as your physicality permits.

Of all the running tests the 1.5-mile is probably the trickiest. It sits in this physiological grey area between the aerobic and anaerobic energy systems. Consequently, if you start too fast, your legs quickly fill with led-like lactate before covering the first quarter. But by erring on the side of caution, and maintaining a methodical pace, your time will only ever be substandard. Thus, for the 1.5-mile, strategy is everything.

To achieve the best possible personal time on this fitness test you must remain as close as you dare to your aerobic threshold (85% of maximum heart rate – ±5%). From the first to the final metre the pace poses a constant challenge to maintain.

A respectable time for the 1.5-mile would be 10-minutes or under. Sub-eight-minutes is excellent and sub 7:30 is exceptional. (These times are based on military attainment: elite fighting units, such as the Royal Marine Commandos or Parachute Regiment, require a prospective recruit to cover the distance in 9:20.)

When considering times for certain running distances (5k, 10k, half/full marathon) it is perhaps best to focus our attention more on pacing. A 6-minute mile pace is to runners what a 20mph/average is to cyclists – that is, a coveted benchmark that indicates superior athletic performance. The further away from this benchmark pace (6-minute mile) the slower your time in whichever distance you are testing yourself over.

10-mile cycle time trial

The 10-mile time trial is ubiquitously used as a means of measuring a cyclist's cardiovascular capacity and power outputs. It is to cyclists what the 1.5-mile is to runners – that is, a challenging high-intensity short distance test that hurts from the first to the very last metre.

For the duration of the distance the cyclist, if he or she harbours any real hope of achieving a good time, must maintain an aerobic output perilously close to the upper maximum; a watt or two away from triggering the anaerobic energy system and slipping into oxygen debt.

It's for this reason that a thorough warm-up is an essential and indispensable preparatory prerequisite of this test.

Before we willingly subject ourselves to between 25- and 35-minutes of sustained suffering, we need to ensure that our physiological systems are adequately prepared for the demands of the test.

The best method of approach for the 10-mile time trial is quite simple. Once sufficiently warmed up we would quickly climb to our target pace. From here on out our objective is to hold this pace for as long as physically possible. It is only over the final mile when we would consider increasing the pace, perhaps sprinting for the line if the legs haven't melted to jelly.

If you fancy having a bash at this test the current world record for the 10-mile time trial stands at 16:35 – which is a little shy of 40-miles per hour!

Muscular endurance tests

A trainer who is said to have good muscular endurance is one who can exert force against a resistance for extended periods. In a single exposure (or set) he or she performs multiple repetitions of an exercise – such as press-ups or pull-ups – without rest or pause.

It is not uncommon for people to confuse muscular endurance with strength. This is not surprising when we take into consideration that one trainer could perform an exercise with ease whereas another might struggle to perform the same exercise for a single rep.

I've always found this to be case with pull-ups. Having helped prepare young people physically for military service, which requires that the prospective recruit comfortably perform multiple 'heaves', I've often found myself shocked at the tremendous disparity in abilities. What can be for some students a relatively easy exercise can for others be an almost insurmountable Herculean labour.

The reason why I mention this is because it is the trainer's physicality that ultimately determines if a resistance exercise is either muscular endurance or strength.

However, so as to set the two apart, I have identified a number of characteristics that are synonymous with muscular endurance training.

- High repetitions that exceed 12
- The resistance is light
- The period of time the exercise spans ranges from 30-seconds to 1-minute (but could easily exceed this upper limit)
- The repetitions are performed in a smooth unbroken continuous movement with no noticeable breaks or pauses

2-minute press-up test

The 2-minute press-up test is used throughout the British military to assess a recruit's muscular endurance. In one long line recruits will be ordered to adopt the press-up position while a partner lies on the floor at their front, arm stretched out and hand clenched into a fist directly under their chest.

On command of the Physical Training Instructor (PTI), the recruit will be given the order to perform as many press-ups as possible in two-minutes. The partner, who looks away, only counts a repetition when they feel the chest of the recruit performing the press-ups make contact with their fist. No contact, no rep.

Though this method is not in the least scientific and transgresses VRR, it does provide PTIs with an insight into a recruit's muscular endurance capacity. Furthermore, it is an indicator of prior practice – if a recruit can only perform, say, 10 repetitions, then they clearly haven't adequately prepared for the rigours of military basic training – and establishes a physical start point from which to chart progression.

If you decide to use the 2-minute press-up test as means of measuring muscular endurance, there are several points you ought to take into consideration. For example:

1. Solicit the services of a second to monitor a) the quality of your repetitions and b) the number of repetitions performed. (Prior to starting the test, it is best to first agree on what constitutes a quality repetition – and ensure that you can use the same person come retest.)
2. For pacing purposes ask the second to keep you informed of the passage of time – either every 20- or 30-seconds that elapses. This intervention will better enable you to budget your energy as you progress through the test.
3. Prior to conducting the test decide your plan of approach. If you rarely perform press-ups, I advise sticking to reps of two or five interspersed with brief rest periods. This will slow the onset of muscle fatigue.
4. Hand positioning: the hands should be positioned in line with the chest and slightly over shoulder-width.
5. Position a soft object of about four deep directly under your chest. For a repetition to constitute as such you must touch the object. It goes without saying that the same object should be used when you retest.

To achieve a good score on the 2-minute press-up test you should aim to exceed 50 full repetitions. The elite military units – Royal Marine Commandos and Parachute Regiment – require that prospective recruits to achieve 55 or more. This attainment is made more challenging by the strict stipulation that at no point during the test can recruits rest on their knees.

For those who are using this test as a means of measuring muscular endurance, and not for military pre-selection training, emphasis ought to be placed on the improvement made from the initial test to the retest.

If you only managed to score five reps in two-minutes during the initial test, but advance that by 10 or more two weeks later, physical development has been made. Such positive feedback is not only suggestive of an effective exercise programme but serves to boost motivation which in turn improves training consistency. These outcomes are testament to the importance of adopting the fitness testing ethos.

Strength test

Strength is defined as 'the maximum force that can be developed during muscular contraction' (Watson 1995). We say someone is strong if they can lift a heavy load or perform physical feats that few could – such as a gymnast holding the crucifix, an Olympic lifter snatching 200 kilograms, or a strongman heaving half a car above their head.

However, a real show of strength is not necessarily indicated by how much weight can be moved during a single contraction. A better means of measuring strength is how much of one's body weight can be moved in a single contraction.

If a strength athlete weighing 100kg can squat 200kg, are they stronger than the athlete who weighs 60kg but can squat 150kg? Yes, the first athlete can lift 50kg more. However, when expressed as a percentage of their body weight, they are in fact lifting less. Thus, pound-for-pound the lighter athlete possesses greater strength.

One-repetition max (1RM)

The 1RM is the go-to test for ascertaining strength. After selecting a compound exercise – squat, deadlift, bent-over row, bench press – the trainer will begin the process of establishing their 1RM by using lighter lifts as steppingstones to their maximal poundage.

To conduct this test, then, you would first decide which compound exercise you wish to establish your 1RM on. Prior to initiating the series of lighter lifts, it is preferable to have a perceived 1RM that you can progress towards.

If you have never attempted this test before and you are clueless as to what your 1RM is, select a weight with which you can perform five repetitions. From this weight proceed to establish your 1RM. Remember: you are only performing one repetition with each lift.

Below I have outlined a number of points that should be taken into consideration prior to attempting the 1RM strength test.

- Ensure to have a second to support and spot you through the lift. Depending on the compound exercise you choose, the 1RM can be dangerous to do on your own (this is especially so with the bench press and squat). Remember, safety first!
- Make sure that you are thoroughly warmed up prior to attempting the test.
- Take long rest periods between lifts (3- to 5-minutes).
- If possible, conduct the test away from other gym users for the following reasons: a) you do not want to be disturbed or distracted during a maximal lift; b) you do not want someone knocking into you; c) if for any reason the weight must be dropped, it's best not to do so on that unsuspecting person to your left performing the plank.
- Increase the weight incrementally – 5kg/2.5kg/1¼kg.
- Leave your ego at the gym door!

Other fitness tests
- **12-minute Cooper run** (cardiovascular): the subject aims to cover the greatest possible distance in 12-minutes. Typically, the Cooper run is conducted on a track or flat open space such as a sports field. However, it can be performed on a treadmill.

- **Vertical jump test** (anaerobic power): the subject attempts to propel themselves as high off the floor as possible in a single explosive movement.
- **30-second Wingate test** (anaerobic power): over a 30-second exposure the subject attempts to exert as much force against an ergometer as possible. Think Chris Hoy during a sprint (who apparently could exert over 2500 watts – which is colossal).
- **Maximum oxygen uptake**: aims to determine the maximum oxygen uptake of the subject while he or she engages in a cardiovascular exercise – usually running on a treadmill at 10% incline.
- **Heart rate (HR) max test**: the aim of this test is to establish the subject's maximum heart rate. It is helpful to know our maximum heart rate because only then are we able to calculate the upper limits of our aerobic threshold and, if we plan on adopting a more scientific approach to our training, it allows us to create a rate of self-perceived exertion (RPE) scale that isn't judged solely off subjective interpretation. To carry out this test begin exercising – running, cycling, rowing – at a medium to high intensity, and over four to 10-minutes gradually increase the intensity until you cannot carry on. It is at this point that you should record your heart rate (Shepherd 2006).

To Conclude

In this workout I've endeavoured to bring your attention to the importance of cultivating an appetite for fitness testing. This practice ought to be habituated as part of your general training routine. For the benefits of fitness testing will only be conferred if they are conducted regularly.

Additionally, to help you improve the accuracy of your test results, a testing procedure based on *validity, reliability,* and *replicability* (VRR) has been produced. Though by no means infallible, observing this procedure will improve testing accuracy. Remember, the results obtained from a poorly conducted test can distort and mislead comprehension concerning our current state of physicality. (Think about that acquaintance of mine who was under the delusion that he could row a sub-five-minute 2000m ergo row.)

And, finally, I have included a comprehensive range of fitness tests that you can use as means of assessing current fitness levels and monitoring performance over time. The aim of this workout is not so much to provide you with the means of testing – for there are many books out there that do a much better job than this one – but to kindle your courage and confidence to have a go.

Workout 42
10,000 Kettlebell Swing Challenge

Swinging isn't just a seedy pastime for the depraved and/or people who have become bored in their relationship. Swinging, if it involves a kettlebell, is a tremendous exercise that promotes a bewildering array of physiological adaptations. Some of the fitness benefits ascribed to kettlebell swinging include:

- Augmented whole-body fitness
- Cast iron posterior chain development (the posterior chain includes the hamstrings, gluteus maximus, and muscles of the lower back)
- Gorilla-like grip strength
- Enhanced aerobic fitness
- Improved muscular endurance
- Improved posture
- Improved body composition – translation: reduced fat mass and increased fat-free mass

Turning our attention from the exercise to the tool itself, kettlebells make for brilliant training equipment because they take up hardly any space, are extremely versatile (I've heard it said that there are over 25 different exercises that can be performed with a single bell!), and they are almost indestructible. It's for these reasons – and more left unmentioned – why they've been dubbed an all-in-one gym.

Right, now we know that the kettlebell swing is a killer exercise, and that the kettlebell is a piece of training equipment par excellence, it makes ruddy good sense to undertake this challenge. But first a few questions need asking . . . then answering.

What is the 10,000 kettlebell swing challenge? And which sadist conceived it?

I'll answer the latter first. Dan John, fitness author, former Olympic athlete, and strength and conditioning coach, conceived of this challenge because, in his words, 'it's one of the simplest – and maybe the best – home training programs [and] it provides results, challenges you, and, most importantly, doesn't suck.'

And in answer to the former question, the 10,000 kettlebell swing challenge involves completing 500 swings a day for 20 consecutive days.

What fitness benefits you can expect from undertaking the challenge?

According to the progenitor of the 10,000 rep challenge – Dan John – you may enjoy one or more of the following fitness benefits:

1: Improved body composition. It's a no-brainer, 10,000 kettlebell swings over 20 days will consume a hell of a lot of calories. And it's going to burn those calories while also promoting the growth of lean muscle mass. Thus, throughout this challenge, we can expect our fat percentage to decrease while simultaneously experiencing an increase in the size and density of our muscle tissue. These highly coveted outcomes will be compounded if you continue with your pre-established training regime (during the challenge!) and maintain a healthy diet.

2: Increased muscle definition. Before Dan John bequeathed the world with this bell swinging behemoth, he enlisted a team of lab rats to test it on. Prior to embarking on the swingathon, each member of the team was weighed and measured. Apparently, to quote Dan John, at the end of 20 days 'Every lifter who was tested after this challenge increased lean muscle mass and conditioning.' It'd of course come more of a surprise if those lifters hadn't experienced a noticeable bump in muscle mass and conditioning. However, so long as you select a suitable bell weight, and you complete all 10,000 swings ensuring to stick to the prescribed 500 reps a day for 20 days, then you almost certainly will increase lean muscle mass and conditioning.

3: Feel good factor. You'll be imbued with a sense of achievement and accomplishment as you will be one of the few people who started the challenge and completed it. (That positive outcome is contingent on you overcoming two huge hurdles. Hurdle one: you do decide to undertake the challenge. Hurdle two: you maintain discipline and motivation enough to emerge victorious.)

4: Develop surgical swinging skills. Be it rep one or rep 9,991, you'll certainly improve – nay! *perfect* – your kettlebell swing technique. Concluding the challenge, you should be a veritable swinging god and even pass off as a seasoned Russian Girevoy competitor!

But there are even more benefits to be had!

Revisiting Dan John's team of lab rats, while working through the 10,000 reps they intermittently met up and reported both their experiences and physiological adaptations. Below is a succinct encapsulation of some of those reported experiences and adaptations:

- ✓ Improved muscle definition
- ✓ Dropping of waist sizes
- ✓ Increased grip strength
- ✓ Noticeable body compositional improvements
- ✓ Augmentation of pre-existing lean muscle mass
- ✓ Enhanced energy levels
- ✓ Advancements of strength PBs
- ✓ Body strength 'shot through the roof'
- ✓ Abs really did take on the appearance of slabs!
- ✓ Boosted training focus and motivation

How to approach the challenge

As the saying goes, there's more than one way to complete 10,000 kettlebell swings. Actually, there are three, each of which has been briefly outlined and explained below.

Way One) The first approach is by far the simplest: it matters not a jot how you do it, how many sets, how many reps, how long you rest, the time of day, etc., etc. . . . just swing that damn bell 500 times every day for 20 days! That, in a nutshell, is way one.

Way Two) Before you bother to read this one you ought to be aware that this way will only work for those who are well endowed with bells. Here's how it works: line up, say, ten kettlebells (Dan John recommends mixing the poods), and, starting at one end, proceed to perform 10 repetitions.

Once you've polished off your 10 reps take one step to the left (or right) and do the same again until you have progressed down the line of bells. If you use the same numerical system as I do, that'll be 100 reps deposited in the kitty. Another four times through and you'll have earned 500 big ones!

Way Three) Now, of the three ways, this one is the most complicated. The daily target of 500 reps is broken down into four sets of 100 reps which again is broken into another four sets – and no, if you assumed this was going to follow some sort of numerical logic, not into clusters of 25 reps. The four sets that will amount to 100 reps are organised as follows:

Set 1: 10 reps
Set 2: 15 reps
Set 3: 25 reps
Set 4: 50 reps

Why so seemingly an arbitrary assortment of rep ranges? Couldn't tell you to be perfectly honest. However, the original challenge – which we'll call 10,000 Kettlebell Swing Challenge 1.0 – included other exercises which were supposed to be performed between each set. Those other exercises include barbell press, dips, goblet squats, and pull-ups. As I understand it, you are to interchange through the four exercises each day. See interchange and rep range example below:

Monday

Set 1: 10 reps (KBS)

1 barbell press

Set 2: 15 reps

2 barbell presses

Set 3: 25 reps

3 barbell presses

Set 4: 50 reps

Rest 30 – 60-seconds

Repeat four more times through. Total swings: 500. Total barbell presses: 30.

Tuesday

Set 1: 10 reps (KBS)

1 dip

Set 2: 15 reps

2 dips

Set 3: 25 reps

3 dips

Set 4: 50 reps

Rest 30 – 60-seconds

Repeat four more times through. Total swings: 500. Total dips: 30.

Got it? Good! Now it's up to you to decide which one of the three ways will best enable you to tackle those 10,000 reps. I opted for way three because, quite simply, it poses the greater challenge. Plus, those additional exercises serve to attenuate the monotony of 500 daily swings.

Vital statistics

Below I have tabulated and calculated various metrics that together showcase what a mammoth challenge stands before you. Personally, I find it motivational knowing, say, how many hundreds of thousands of kilograms I'll lift and shift throughout a challenge, or how many miles I'll cover over the course of a competition. If you're like-minded, then the post-challenge totals that follow will whet your appetite for this Herculean labour. However, if you're hungry to start swinging, flick forward to the challenge calendar located in the workout conclusion.

Total weight lifted

In the original challenge outline, Dan John advises women to use a 16kg kettlebell and men a 24kg. By following these advisory weights women would, after completing all 10,000 repetitions, lift a combined total of 160,000kg (160 tons) and men 240,000kg (240 tons). That's some going.

You might be wondering how I arrived at these obscene total figures? Simple! Every swing constitutes as one times the weight lifted. So, if you swing a 16kg kettlebell once, you have 'lifted' or 'shifted' or 'swung' 16kg. I doubt anyone could refute that slice of logic. Now, if you completed a set of 10 swings you merely multiply the weight by the number of swings: 10 x 16 = 160(kg). You with me? Ok, good. By scaling the multiplication integer up to 10,000 and sticking in front of it whatever weight bell you swung, you will very quickly arrive at your overall poundage. (The training method of kilogram accumulation is explained more fully in Appendix A.)

I opted for a 32kg and, on a couple of occasions, a 40kg kettlebell. However, interchanging between the two weights as I did, made calculating the total poundage a tad tricky. But after a spot of numerical gymnastics, I arrived at a rather pleasing total of 344,000kg.

Total distance covered

In addition to shifting a shedload of weight, you'll also cover some serious ground without even taking a single step. Let me explain that cryptic opener.

For reasons unknown, I get a kick out of calculating every aspect of my training sessions. This inveterate pedantic predisposition seeped into this challenge and, while out on an evening stroll, I thought it'd be a good idea to measure the distance the kettlebell would travel after being swung 10,000 times.

This is how I worked out the distance.

I stood next to a whiteboard and, armed with an unsheathed marker pen, proceeded to perform a swing thus tracing out the arc that the kettlebell will follow 20,000 times. (Did you say 20,000 times? Yes! Remember: what goes up must come down. And though that is two separate directions it still only constitutes as one repetition.) I then tacked a piece of string over the arc and measured the string.

In my intellectually impoverished mind, this was the most accurate and effective way to calculate the distance the kettlebell would travel with each swing. I'm sure the closet Kurt Gödel could conceive a more logical method (email me if you do).

The crude measuring method outlined above showed that the kettlebell, on completion of each swing, travelled 7 feet 4 inches (or 88 inches, or 224cm). To calculate the total distance, I merely multiplied 7'4" by 10,000. Of course, this resulted in a ridiculous figure of 73,333 feet. Which means precisely nothing in real money. But when calculated into a comprehendible distance it transpired that I moved the kettlebell about 24 kilometres. (Though this figure is almost certainly incorrect – where's Jordan Ellenberg when you need him!)

Total time taken
And finally, I timed how long I spent swinging across the 20 days. In total, the 10,000 swings took me 5-hours, 11-minutes, and 29-seconds to complete. Although, I'm inclined to include a caveat. And that is, that time is inaccurate.

A closer chronological account would see it somewhere around 5-hours and 30-minutes. Why the discrepancy? Some days I'd get so absorbed swinging my bell that I'd forget to start the timer. Also, my chronometer – as technology is apt to – let me down on more than one occasion and so I had to guestimate.

However, irrespective of my laissez-faire experimental approach, I still arrived at a reasonably accurate time.

Kettlebell swing tutorial

Before attempting this challenge, I highly advise that you spend a few days – or even a week – working on your swing technique. For it would be a big mistake to complete 10,000 repetitions of an exercise that you are performing incorrectly. Of course, by doing so you will not only make your life harder, perhaps by dipping too low on the downwards phase (the most common mistake), but, of primary concern, you will increase injury susceptibility. So, with that said, get your swing in good order before you set sail on this Odyssey.

The step-by-step teaching points below will provide you with a comprehensive overview of how to perform a kettlebell swing correctly. Once you nail down the basics spend some time working on your form.

Teaching points

As exercise names go the kettlebell swing couldn't be less ambiguous if it tried. After taking the kettlebell from the floor with both hands we initiate the movement with a short backward pull then thrust forwards through the hips propelling that gravity-loving lump of pig iron level with our shoulders.

Congratulations! You are now a certified swinger!

But wait, don't go anywhere yet. If you've never swung before, ensure to familiarise yourself with the following list of teaching points. Though an indubitably simple exercise there are several technical considerations that, well, you ought to consider.

1. Centre your mass over a kettlebell the weight of which is commensurate with your current strength and ability. In short, don't go heavy, keep it light to begin with.
2. Bending at the knee while ensuring to keep the back ironing-board straight, grasp the bell with both hands.
3. Firing through the quads squat into the standing position.

4. Before initiating the movement organise your feet – they should be just over shoulder-width apart – fix your eyes on an indefinite point in the distance and prepare your mind for the exercise.
5. With knees still slightly bent rotate slightly at the hips so as to create space to pull the bell back between your pins.
6. On receiving the kettlebell in your groin, fire through with the gluteal muscles and, with arms straight, propel the bell forward. Instead of trying to get the KB level with your shoulders in the first swing, I find it best to elevate it in stages. Usually, after the third swing, I'm in full flight.
7. Once the kettlebell has reached the desired height – roughly level with your chin – arrest the movement and allow gravity to do its thing. Ensure to control the kettlebell during its descent.
8. Again, receive the KB in the groin harnessing the kinetic energy generated.
9. Use that energy (and a bit of your own) to complete the next repetition.
10. *Now* you are swinging!

Swinging dos
✓ Keep control throughout the exercise
✓ Relax during the movement – you shouldn't strike the appearance of a soldier on parade
✓ Make sure that your feet are evenly spaced and planted firmly before attempting the swing
✓ Fix your eyes on a point roughly head height
✓ Ensure the arms are slightly bent throughout
✓ Keep your core tight while swinging
✓ Squeeze your bum cheeks together at precisely the moment when the KB reaches the top position. It helps to imagine that you are trying to crack a walnut between your arse cheeks.

Swinging don'ts
⊗ Do not bend or round your back – keep it straight or slightly concaved
⊗ Do not at any point lock the legs out

⊗ Do not over-rotate or 'collapse' at the hips during the downward phase. The kettlebell should not pull you down so that your torso becomes parallel with the floor. This is a common mistake that places a lot of stress on the lumbar region of the spine.

Five lessons learned after 10,000 swings

On concluding any challenge or undertaking it is prudent practice to apprise personal performance. Adopting this ethos enables us to identify areas where we can improve while illuminating areas worthy of recognition and commendation. Legend has it that the great Greek geometrician Pythagoras exhorted his adherents to reflect on everything they did. 'Do not sleep until you have examined every action of the day.'

Following in Pythagoras' philosophical footsteps, I've endeavoured to outline in brief five lessons learned after 10,000 kettlebell swings. Though informal and largely superfluous, the lessons identify barriers and hurdles that I had to surmount on my journey through this gruelling challenge. But what's of potential use to you, dear reader, is the methods and strategies I employed to overcome those barriers and hurdles.

As it is likely that you will encounter the same problems, the scattered reflections below will equip you with the means of extrication should you find yourself in a similar funk.

Lesson #1: It's good to work with others when undertaking an arduous ordeal.
A couple of days before smashing a champagne bottle against the hull of my 32kg kettlebell and launching it on the wild and wasteful ocean in search of that infamous White Whale, I asked a couple of training pals if they'd like to accompany me on the voyage of 10,000 swings. Unsurprisingly, they all flatly declined.

So, I put the prospect to the only person I knew who possessed a pair of bells. When I got down on one knee before my much better half and proposed the challenge she instantly – without a moment's hesitation – proclaimed 'Yes!' And on that day, we started swinging together.

I must admit that working with someone through this challenge made swinging that bell a lot less banal. Whenever motivation or enthusiasm waned, we would encourage each other to continue on swinging. And during our daily dose of 500 reps, we'd sometimes swing in tandem or take turns, motivating each other through a set of 100 reps.

Lesson #2: When the going gets tough you've just gotta keep on swinging regardless. By doing so you'll almost certainly succeed.
Being the egotist that I am, I scoffed a Dan John's recommendation to use a 24kg KB and instead opted for 32kg. Now, if you've ever used a traditional Girevoy competition kettlebell, you'll know that the handles are designed to accommodate one hand – not two. Also, the handles are thin and often abrasive.

These design features are not necessarily a problem when performing classical single-handed exercises – such as the snatch, jerk, clean, and so on. However, when you squeeze a second hand into that small space, your fingers inevitably crunch and crimp together somewhat like the way sardines are in a tin.

The consequence? After the first set of 500 swings, a number of nasty blisters and sores started forming along the lengths of my fingers. An inauspicious start to the challenge. Especially considering that one of those blisters eventually turned gangrenous which resulted in the surgical removal of several digits. I'm just pulling your bell.

But, irrespective of the thankful fact that those blisters didn't result in an amputation, they – the blisters – certainly put a sting in the swing. And after that very first set, with 9,500 swings still hanging in the balance, I knew that I would have to muster the full force of my internal resolve to see this challenge through to fruition.

The going got tough but I got that bit tougher. If you dare pit your physicality and psychology against this challenge, I can guarantee that you will at some point have to do the same. Be prepared for this.

Lesson #3: Adapt and overcome!
This is an old Royal Marine maxim that, after years of inculcation, has been permanently branded in my brain. It probably traces its origins to Darwin's oft misquoted axiom that it's not the strongest species that survive, it's the species most *adaptable* to change.

However, irrespective of who coined the phrase – Darwin or the Royal Marines – it still serves as a source of sound advice when an insurmountable wall stands in your way. What I'm trying to say here is, if for whatever reason you find Dan John's prescriptive method to be incompatible with your training preferences and feel that it may adversely impact your prospects of emerging victorious from the challenge, there's no rule against modifying or adapting it.

For example, I much preferred to descend the rep range from 50 down to 10 as opposed to starting at 10 and climbing up to 50. A psychological thing. Also, I often merged the 15 and 10 rep sets together. This, I found, not only speeded things along a little but took the sting out of the next set of swings. And finally, instead of resting for a minute on completion of each 100 reps, I hopped on the rower and completed 1000m at a gingerly pace (see typical session layout below). Rowing aided recovery and made what is essentially a warm-up into a worthwhile training session as well as mitigating the monotony of swinging that bell 500 times.

So, by adapting the challenge, I not only overcame it but bettered my physicality in the process.

Typical session
2000m row warm-up
50 swings (32kg)

5 no-weight squats
25 swings (32kg)
4 no-weight squats
15 swings (32kg)
3 no-weight squats
10 swings (32kg)
1000m row
Repeat four more times.

Lesson #4: Flawless form isn't an option, it's a categorical imperative!

The necessary importance of applying perfect form when exercising is not only incontestable – who's going to waste their time with a refutation? – but is an indomitable axiom to which all fitness professionals faithfully adhere and zealously propound. Ever heard a personal trainer tell their client to round their back when deadlifting? Or lockout at the knee when squatting? Could you even imagine such a situation? Most certainly not!

The application of proper form (or technique) becomes increasingly important when the weight gets heavier and the rep range gets greater. Yes, of course, it's true that we run the risk of injury even when applying poor form during a light lift. However, heavy weights and high reps not only increase injury susceptibility but also (potentially) compound the severity of the injury. Thus, it is imperative that, when engaging in resistance exercise, we pay close attention to the quality of our form ensuring always to observe safe lifting principles.

This advice, though seemingly tautological, tends to flee the mind when it's most needed. Which was the case one morning during the challenge when I unthinkingly hoisted my 32kg KB off the floor with a rounded back. Tut, tut, tut!

At first, I thought I felt something go at the base of my spine, which put the scarers in me. But after tentatively trying to locate what I assumed to be a pulled muscle, I was mightily relieved to discover that no such misfortune had befallen me.

However, having escaped unscathed, I made a generous libation to the training Gods and repented by paying extra attention to my form. Before the end of the challenge, I'd perfected – from pick up to put down – every inch of the swing technique.

I advise that you perfect your swing prior to initiating the challenge. See the technique tutorial above.

Lesson #5: The power of persistence.
I won't try to mislead the reader by painting a colourful picture of my performance. I'll tell it how it is (was). This challenge gets mind-numbingly boring and completing those 500 swings induces a Groundhogian Day monotony. I'm non-too ashamed to admit that, before reaching the halfway point, I was seriously flirting with the idea of throwing in the bell.

Plus, a nasty rigor mortis-like cramp-cum-arthritis settled in two of the fingers of my left hand. Normally I'd simply shrug such a problem off and crack on regardless. However, I'm an avid guitarist and wouldn't jeopardise that guilty pleasure for a purposeless challenge.

But the ego in me wanted to finish. For I would not be able to hold my head high among the fictitious crowd of spectators that I'd conjured in my mind – who clap and cheered my every swing. Also, the insidious integrity in me, a hereditary affliction, wouldn't allow me to publish this workout had I not completed the challenge to the exact specifications laid out by its progenitor.

So, I did a spot of remedial on my stiff appendages, spiced up the swing sessions by including some rowing and boxing, and persevered until all 10,000 reps had been banked.

Positive post-challenge outcomes
- I can now swing a 32kg KB with the comfort and ease that I previously could a 24kg KB.

- I noticed posterior chain strength gains which translated into improved performance in other disciplines.
- The augmentation in grip and forward-thrusting strength enabled me to advance my 10k rowing PB by half a second per 500m.
- A corollary of the previous point, it made carrying the weekly shopping a hell of a lot easier.
- Those 10,000 swings acted like a hammer and anvil to my transverse abdominus and on completion of the challenge, my abs were not only more defined but rock solid.
- I maintained sufficient discipline, dedication, and determination to complete the challenge. And though the feat of swinging a kettlebell 10,000 times over 20 days is not on par with, say, completing an Ironman or cycling the Tour de France, which very nearly spans the same number of days, it still required that rarely seen quality that goes by the name of *commitment*. Due to my jam-packed lifestyle and my obstinate refusal to stop participating in my pre-established exercise regime, at least 5,000 swings were performed before 5 am.
- I experienced augmented pulling power – and not the type of pulling polygamists pursue. A week or so after the challenge I had a crack at my obligatory bi-monthly 15,000m row, which I try to complete in under an hour (2:00/500 = exactly one-hour). To do so can be a bit of a barney. However, I was pleasantly surprised at how effortless I found this distance after the challenge. So effortless in fact that I rowed on to 21,097 (a half marathon) sustaining the same pace.

Conclusion

Stop reading 'n get swinging!

10,000 Kettlebell Swing Challenge Calendar

Day 1	Day 2	Day 3	Day 4	Day 5	Day 6	Day 7
500 – 32kg	500 – 32kg	500 – 40kg	500 – 32kg	500 – 40kg	500 – 40kg	500 – 32kg
T: 14:09	T: 13:46	T: 14:49	T: 16:09	T: 15:51	T: 16:03	T: 14:26
	27:55	42:44	58:53	1:14:44	1:30:47	1:45:13
Day 8	**Day 9**	**Day 10**	**Day 11**	**Day 12**	**Day 13**	**Day 14**
500 – 32kg	500 – 32kg	500 – 32kg	500 – 32kg	500 – 32kg	500 – 32kg	500 – 32kg
T: 15:09	T: 17:12	T: 15:01	T: 16:21	T: 15:41	T: 16:36	T: 15:58
2:00:22	2:17:34	2:32:35	2:48:56	3:04:37	3:21:13	3:37:11
Day 15	**Day 16**	**Day 17**	**Day 18**	**Day 19**	**Day 20**	Finish!
500 – 32kg	500 – 32kg	500 – 32kg	500 – 32kg	500 – 32kg	500 – 32kg	
T: 14:42	T: 15:07	T: 16:23	T: 16:45	T: 15:58	T: 15:43	
3:51:53	4:07:00	4:23:23	4:40:08	4:56:06	5:11:29	

Workout 43
Train Like a Martial Arts Legend

If you want to develop insane strength and sculpt a super-chiselled physique, you must start training like a martial arts master. The two workouts below were developed by Bruce Lee to help him forge his legendary physicality.

Comprised of exercise elements from a wide range of training methods, Lee designed the workouts to build whole-body strength, muscular endurance while also increasing aerobic fitness.

According to John Little, who compiled Lee's workouts and routines in the brilliant book *The Art of Expressing the Human Body*, 'Not long after discovering the benefits to be attained from proper bodybuilding and strength training, Bruce Lee decided that he should balance his muscular development and strength by subjecting each muscle group of the body to progressive-resistance training.'

It was from this discovery that Lee began the process of formulating the following fitness sessions.

Bruce Lee's workout ethos

Bruce Lee believed in achieving physical excellence through persistent hard work and dedication. This fact is evidenced in his personal training diaries which document a five-hour a day training routine.

He also knew that to improve you must keep pushing beyond your perceived physical limitations. Lee made this patently clear to a training partner while out on a run.

'So we get to three, we go into the fourth mile and . . . then I really begin to give out. "Bruce if I run anymore . . . I'm liable to have a heart attack and die." He said, "Then die." It made me so mad that I went the full five miles.'

When after the run the training partner asked, "Why did you say that?" Bruce retorted:

'If you always put limits on what you can do, physical or anything else, it'll spread into the rest of your life. It'll spread into your work, into your morality, into your entire being . . . There are no limits. There are plateaus, but you must not stay there, you must go beyond them.'

Bruce Lee's training approach

Though an unabashed taskmaster, Bruce Lee understood the importance of training safely. Yes, we should push ourselves. Yes, we should strive to go beyond plateaus. However, correct form must precede all other training priorities.

'Above all else,' Lee tells us, 'never cheat on an exercise; use the amount of weight that you can handle without undue strain.'

For Bruce, this lesson was learned the hard way. While performing good mornings with a 70kg Olympic barbell, Lee suffered a devastating lower back injury. From this training accident, which he later attributed to applying unnecessary resistance, Lee was left confined to an armchair for six-months. His attending physician informed him that he might never walk again, let alone become a martial arts master.

Of course, we all know that Bruce proved the doctor's prognosis wrong.

Exercise experimentation

Working hard and safely were two pillars of Bruce Lee's training methodology. Another key aspect of his pursuit of physical excellence was the experimentation with contemporary exercise approaches.

Lee was always testing and trialling different training regimes, refining his workouts, and augmenting his repertoire of exercises. He even commissioned a metalsmith to manufacture training tools of his own design.

In addition to forging a robust physicality through exercise experimentation, Lee was an advocate of balance. Above all, 'he wanted harmony among all muscle groups so they could generate power in concert, and would combine to accomplish a single objective' – that is, to be more effective in combat (*The Art of Expressing the Human Body*).

Bruce Lee's dos and don'ts of training
✓ Do a complete extension and contraction
✓ Do all exercises at a reasonable speed to keep the muscles warm
⊗ Don't cheat on any exercise
⊗ Don't lift more weight than you can handle without undue strain

Bruce Lee workout benefits

The workouts below will help you to develop strength and general fitness. In designing these workouts Lee applied learning and experimentation to maximise the effectiveness of the combination of exercises.

Comprised of big compound movements, Lee's General Development Routine engages the major muscle groups. Thus, even though the workout is short, it still provides a whole-body training session. And because it can be approached as an AMRAP or HIIT, the General Development Routine has the capacity to stimulate the cardiovascular system.

But if you opt purely for the strength approach, that's fine. The second workout was designed specially to enhance aerobic capacity.

Lee's Total Fitness Routine, as he aptly christened it, which is essentially circuit training, focuses on aerobic fitness and physical dynamism. Comprised exclusively of cardio and calisthenics, this workout is a great whole-body conditioner that will also burn fat and improve muscle definition.

Interchanging between the two training sessions will deliver a powerful fitness punch. For example, you could make the General Development Routine your Tuesday and Thursday whole-body strength-building blast and the Total Fitness Routine your Monday, Wednesday, and Friday complete conditioning kick.

Do this and you might stand a fighting chance of achieving an ounce of Lee's physical supremacy.

Warm-up

Prior to completing Bruce Lee's workouts, spend 10-minutes warming up first. Skipping or rowing are excellent warm-up exercises as they engage the major muscle groups. Also, to prepare the muscles for resistance training, include three to five sets of light exercises from the routine.

Bruce Lee's General Development Routine

Lee's General Development Routine was designed to 'balance his muscular development and strength.' It is comprised of eight exercises all of which were completed with a barbell.

The set and rep ranges in Lee's original plan are suggestive of a mix of strength and muscular endurance training: two sets of between eight to 12 reps.

However, you don't have to stick to the prescriptive set and rep range. You have the option of making this purely a strength routine by increasing the weight and decreasing the reps – keep the sets around two to three and reps six to 10. For muscular endurance, decrease the weight and increase the sets and reps – three to five and 12 to 20 respectively.

1. Clean and press (2 sets of 8 to 12 reps)
2. Bicep curl (2 sets of 8 to 12 reps)
3. Standing shoulder press (2 sets of 8 to 12 reps)
4. Bent-over row (2 sets of 8 to 12 reps)
5. Barbell squat (2 sets of 8 to 20 reps)
6. Bench press (2 sets of 8 to 12 reps)
7. Barbell pullovers (2 sets of 8 to 12 reps)

Bruce Lee's Total Fitness Routine

Lee tailored the Total Fitness Routine to incorporate the three core training components: cardio, flexibility, and strength. Lee believed that by developing these components in equal measures total fitness could be achieved.

'Training for strength and flexibility is a must. You must use it to support your techniques. Techniques alone are no good if you don't support them with strength and flexibility.'

–Bruce Lee

The Total Fitness Routine is comprised of six one-minute HITs (high-intensity training – no intervals). Your objective is to work as hard as you physically can for each of the six exercises.

In total one round of the routine will take six minutes; there are no rest periods. The great thing about this workout is that it is completely customisable. Meaning, you can shape the number of circuits to suit your time constraints and training requirements. Also, depending on your fitness levels, you can either decrease or increase the exercise intervals.

1. Skipping (1-minute)
2. Burpees (1-minute)
3. Press-ups (1-minute)
4. Star jumps (1-minute)

5. Air squats (1-minute)
6. Plyometric tuck jumps (1-minute)

General advice

- Before attacking Lee's General Development Routine, ensure that you are familiar with all the exercises. I only mention this because the clean and press is a complex movement that requires considerable practice before mastery is achieved. However, in this workout, you do not have to perform the exercise as an Olympic lifter would – that is, observing every minute detail of this multifaceted movement. Instead, you can perform a power clean to push press. Or, if you're not sure how to perform a power clean, you can go deadlift into hang clean into push press. And if you don't know how to do a hang clean, just stick to deadlifting.
- If you've got a fighter's spirit, or you're feeling flushed with energy, consider completing both workouts back-to-back. Combined, you've got a good 20-minutes of exercising here.

Workout 44
Boxing Met-Con Mania

Boxing is the ultimate challenge. There's nothing that can compare to testing yourself the way you do every time you step in the ring.

– Sugar Ray Leonard

This boxing-inspired metabolic conditioning (met-con) workout is the complete training package. The boxing exercise, which is exclusively heavy bag work, will help you build awesome muscular endurance while also enabling you to develop knock-out punching power (whether you want it or not).

The calisthenic exercises, two of which feature dynamic plyometric movements, will improve muscular endurance, explosive power, and impressive muscular tonality. Furthermore, the whole-body resistance exercise adds a strength element to this workout making it a powerful fitness developer.

And finally, the cardio exercise – shuttle sprints – not only improves cardiovascular performance but will also enhance stamina in the legs.

Benefits of boxing training

It's not up for debate, boxing is the ultimate training methodology. If you want to improve all-round fitness, burn fat, increase muscular definition, and sharpen your fighting skills, you've got to take up boxing training.

Of the many forms of exercise available – CrossFit, circuit training, weightlifting, cardio – none engage as many components of fitness as a boxing workout. In a single boxing session – like the one below – your agility, balance, coordination, cardio, power, and muscular endurance will all be tested.

How it works

Organised around a circuit format, this boxing conditioning workout oscillates between the heavy bag and a range of resistance exercises. The mechanics of this session are super simple. When you've completed the warm-up, start at the first exercise – clap-hand press-ups – and aim for as many reps as possible in one-minute. From there, glove up and get straight onto the heavy boxing bag.

Your objective is to maintain high-intensity output for each one-minute round. Once the bell (buzzer) goes you are to transition immediately to the next exercise. After you have completed one full lap of the circuit, that's all 10 exercises, you can take a minute rest.

As soon as your rest is over, get back off your stool, and get back into the fight!

Key points

- Complete the 10-minute warm-up – which is skipping – and throw in a few sets of body weight exercises while you're at it. Burpees are good.
- Concluding the skip (and burpees), set a minute repeat countdown timer.
- Starting at the first exercise, aim to accumulate as many repetitions as possible in the short time allotted.
- Immediately move on to the next exercise.
- Once you have worked through all 10 exercises, take a minute rest.
- When your time's up get straight back into the circuit.
- Repeat for a minimum of three times.

Warm-up

- 10-minutes of skipping interlaced with low intensity body weight exercises.

Workout

💪 Clap-hand press-ups (or normal press-ups if you can't clap)

🥊 **Punchbag** (maintain a high punch output)

💪 Kettlebell swings

🥊 **Punchbag** (maintain a high punch output)

💪 Medicine ball slams

🥊 **Punchbag** (maintain a high punch output)

💪 Sprints (25-metres)

🥊 **Punchbag** (maintain a high punch output)

💪 Box jumps (2-foot)

🥊 **Punchbag** (maintain a high punch output)

General advice

- To make transitioning between exercises easier, gather all the equipment needed near your punching bag. This way when you're done doing a Rocky Balboa breaking the ribs of a cow carcass you can whip off the gloves, reset the timer, and start the next exercise.

- The medicine ball slam, if you're new to this mighty exercise, requires no technical finesse whatsoever. Here's how it works. In one smooth movement you're simply hoisting the ball off the floor and above your head and then, with the wrath of the Raging Bull, slamming it down again between your feet. And if the room isn't shaking and the knees of other trainers quaking, you ain't slamming your ball hard enough!

- *But what if I don't have a punching bag?* Simple, shadowbox instead. To intensify shadowboxing strap yourself into a resistance band or hold hand weights.

This upper body strength workout does more than develop hulk-like strength in the muscles of the back, chest, shoulders, and arms. It explodes muscles endurance while also providing a tough training challenge to sink your teeth into.

In addition to building strength and enhancing muscle endurance, this workout will also increase size in the latissimus dorsi, pectorals, deltoids, and biceps. Furthermore, because this is a high-volume training session, you'll likely enjoy improved muscle definition as well.

How it works

There are two ways that you can tackle this workout. The first is to approach it as you would a typical gym session. Split the workload over a series of sets and implement a rep range suitable for your current level of strength.

We'll call this option one. Below, accompanying the exercise explanations, suggested sets, and rep ranges have been provided.

The second way to approach this workout, which we'll call option two, is to pit yourself against the challenge of lifting 10-ton of weight in the shortest time possible. Option two is in many respects similar to the AMRAP (as many repetitions as possible) training method.

However, the difference here is that your objective is to lift 10-ton as quickly as possible. If you're unfamiliar with this method of training, the process is explained below.

10-ton challenge explained

Calculating your accumulated weight requires scant numerical acumen. Merely multiply the weight being lifted by the number of repetitions performed. Here's an example.

To accrue a combined total lift of 10-ton with, say, a 50kg Olympic barbell, you must perform 200 reps. (Example: 1 rep x 50kg = 50kg lifted. 10 reps x 50kg = 500kg lifted. 200 reps x 50kg = 10,000kg (10-ton) lifted.)

Note: those 200 reps do not have to be performed in one sitting. You can take as long as you need.

Also, the reps should be divided across the four upper body movements. So, you shouldn't need to implement a rest as you'll receive one when transitioning between exercises.

And don't forget to record your time for prosperity. By recording how long it takes to bag that 10-ton, you'll have a benchmark to compete against the next time you have a go at this challenge. This will provide you with a measure to assess physical improvements.

Bundle the exercises into a circuit

One of the most effective ways to approach this challenge is by organising the exercises into a circular circuit. Here's how you could do this:

- Use a single barbell for the exercises as this eradicates the need to chop and change equipment – which wastes time
- Select a weight that you can comfortably lift for 10 reps
- Calculate the number of reps needed to achieve 10-ton for the weight selected
- Stick to 10 reps if possible as it makes calculating the combined weight easier
- Create a tally sheet (or use the examples below) to keep track of your progress
- After a good warm-up, set a timer and start lifting!

Warm-up

Prior to pitting yourself against this workout, irrespective of which option you select, ensure to complete a comprehensive warm. A good 10-minutes of rowing interspersed with light sets of the four exercises should suffice.

Workout

1) Bento-over row

Option 1) strength: 2 to 3 sets of 6 to 10 reps

Option 2) 10-ton challenge: 50 reps of a 50kg barbell = 2500kg

Sets	1	2	3	4	5
Reps	10r	10r	10r	10r	10r

- Hold a barbell at your front; the bar is resting against your quads; palms are facing back.
- Adopt a neutral stance: feet shoulder-width.
- Hinge at the hips until the bar is level with the upper knee.
- Eyes fixed forward, back straight.
- Smoothly row the bar until it touches somewhere between your navel and nips.
- Under control return it to the start position and repeat.

2) Bench press

Option 1) strength: 2 to 3 sets of 6 to 10 reps

Option 2) 10-ton challenge: 50 reps of a 50kg barbell = 2500kg

Sets	1	2	3	4	5
Reps	10r	10r	10r	10r	10r

- Set the barbell at an appropriate height on a rack.

- Manoeuvre a bench under the bar ensuring that it is exactly central.
- Lie on the bench taking a wide grip on the bar.
- Prior to lifting, plant your feet firmly so that your form a stable position to lift from.
- Remove the bar from the rack and lower until it touches the chest.
- Smoothly press the bar to the start position: do not lockout the elbow joint.

3) Hang clean

Option 1) strength: 2 to 3 sets of 6 to 10 reps

Option 2) 10-ton challenge: 50 reps of a 50kg barbell = 2500kg

Sets	1	2	3	4	5
Reps	10r	10r	10r	10r	10r

- Adopt the same start position as outlined for the bent-over row.
- To initiate the hang clean, hinge forward slightly at the hips.
- Using lower back, lat, trap, and arm strength heave the bar up to the shoulders. This should be executed in one fluid movement.
- The bar should be momentarily supported in the front rack position before returning to the start.
- To return the bar to the start position, allow gravity to do the work while you guide and control the bar's descent.
- Of course, a multifaceted movement such as the hang clean is impossible to capture in a written description. But if you observe safe lifting principles, and you're using a light bar, you should avoid catastrophe.

4) Standing shoulder press

Option 1) strength: 2 to 3 sets of 6 to 10 reps

Option 2) 10-ton challenge: 50 reps of a 50kg barbell = 2500kg

Sets	1	2	3	4	5
Reps	10r	10r	10r	10r	10r

- Stand with a bar supported under your chin, hands spaced a little over shoulder-width (aka the top position of the hang clean).
- Your knees are slightly bent.
- You can engage the quads for lift assist if you so wish (this is called a push press).
- To initiate the exercise, press the bar above your head stopping short of lockout.
- Lower under control to the start position in preparedness for the next rep.

General advice

- Ensure that you can safely perform all the exercises before undertaking the workout. Any exercise that you feel uncomfortable performing, replace with one from your stock of favourites.
- To those who plan to step in the ring with the 10-ton challenge, it's wise to draw up a set/rep tally chart before pulling on your gloves. By implementing this advice you'll easily and accurately be able to track progress.
- Another point of note for the 10-ton competitors. The number of sets and reps represented in the trackers have been calculated against a 50kg barbell. If you plan to change the weight (±), you will of course need to recalibrate those reps so that you achieve 2,500kg for each of the four exercises.

Workout 46
10-Ton Lower Body Strength Challenge

This lower body strength workout is the antithesis of its predecessor. Whereas the upper body strength workout was comprised of purely upper body exercises, this lower body . . .

I think you know where I was going with that intro.

One thing I will say, before you set fire to your legs, is that these two workouts can be combined into a Super-Duper Whole Body Strength Workout!

If you decide to merge the two into one *mega sessh!* I advise interlacing the exercises so that you oscillate between upper body/lower body. This will ensure a rest is bestowed on each hemisphere while its geographical opposite is exercising.

Also, for those sadomasochists who dare undertake the 10-ton challenge, remember you'll be doubling the total to 20-ton if you combine the two workouts.

How it works
So, if you completed Workout 45, you already understand how it works and thus can skip straight to the session. However, for those who have taken an arbitrary approach to this book, and are selecting circuits and workouts at random, I've copied the explanation above and pasted it below.

There are two ways that you can tackle this workout. The first is to approach it as you would a typical gym session. Split the workload over a series of sets and implement a rep range suitable for your current level of fitness.

We'll call this option one. Below, accompanying the exercise explanations, suggested sets, and rep ranges have been provided.

The second way to approach this workout, which we'll call option two, is to pit yourself against the challenge of lifting 10-ton of weight in the shortest time possible. Option two is in many respects similar to the AMRAP (as many repetitions as possible) training method.

However, the difference here is that your objective is to lift 10-ton as quickly as possible. If you're unfamiliar with this method of training, the process is explained below.

10-ton challenge explained

Calculating your accumulated weight requires scant numerical acumen. Merely multiply the weight being lifted by the number of repetitions performed. Here's an example.

To accrue a combined total lift of 10-ton with, say, a 50kg Olympic barbell, you must perform 200 reps. (Example: 1 rep x 50kg = 50kg lifted. 10 reps x 50kg = 500kg lifted. 200 reps x 50kg = 10,000kg (10-ton) lifted.)

Note: those 200 reps do not have to be performed in one sitting. You can split them into as many sets as you need.

Also, the reps should be divided across the four leg movements. So, you shouldn't need to implement a rest as you'll receive one when transitioning between exercises.

And don't forget to record your time for prosperity. By recording how long it takes to bag that 10-ton, you'll have a benchmark to compete against the next time you have a go at this challenge. This will provide you with a measure to assess physical improvements against.

Organise the exercise into a circuit

A quick tip: the most effective way to approach this challenge is by organising the exercises into a circuit. Here's how you could do this.

- Use a single barbell for the compound exercises
- Select a weight that you can comfortably lift for 10 reps
- Calculate the number of reps needed to achieve 10-ton on the weight selected
- Stick to 10 reps as it makes calculating the weight easier
- Create a tally sheet (or use the examples below) to keep track of your progress
- After a good warm-up, set a timer and start lifting!

Warm-up

Prior to pitting yourself against this workout, irrespective of which option you select, ensure to complete a comprehensive warm. A good 10-minutes of rowing interspersed with light sets of the four exercises should suffice.

Workout

1) Barbell squat

Option 1) strength: 2 to 3 sets of 6 to 10 reps

Option 2) 10-ton challenge: 50 reps of a 50kg barbell = 2500kg

Sets	1	2	3	4	5
Reps	10r	10r	10r	10r	10r

- With the bar resting securely across your traps, space your feet slightly over shoulder-width apart.
- Keeping your eyes fixed forward, squat down until a 90-degree angle forms at the back of the knee.
- To conclude the squat, stand up under control focusing on pushing your hips forward as you do so.

2) Kettlebell goblet squat

Option 1) strength: 2 to 3 sets of 6 to 10 reps

Option 2) 10-ton challenge: 79 reps of a 32kg kettlebell = 2528kg

Sets	1	2	3	4	5
Reps	15r	15r	15r	15r	19r*

- Stand over a kettlebell with your feet set wider than shoulder-width.
- Grasp the outer edge of the kettlebell handle; your fingers are curled around the handle, your thumbs pointing to the body of the bell.
- Pull the kettlebell back between your legs and upend it.
- If you're in the correct start position, the kettlebell should be suspended level with your chest, arms locked at right angles, and the base of the bell facing the ceiling.
- Squat down until your forearms touch your quads.

3) Dumbbell Farmer's walk

Option 1) strength: 2 to 3 sets of 6 to 10 reps

Option 2) 10-ton challenge: 50-metres of carrying 2 x 25kg dumbbells = 2500kg

Sets	1	2	3	4	5
Reps	10m	10m	10m	10m	10m

- Before breaking into a Farmer's walk, first measure out a 'runway' – that is, a straight walkway that is bereft of obstacles and trip hazards.
- Also, it's good practice to measure the runway so that you know how far you've walked.
- Remember, Farmer's walk is not measured by how many repetitions you perform, but by how many metres you carried a specific load.
- When picking your dumbbells up, ensure to observe correct lifting principles: back straight, tight core, eyes fixed to your front.
- Stand up, compose yourself, and proceed to walk.

4) Overhead squat

Option 1) strength: 2 to 3 sets of 6 to 10 reps

Option 2) 10-ton challenge: 50 reps of a 50kg barbell = 2500kg

Sets	1	2	3	4	5
Reps	10r	10r	10r	10r	10r

As the overhead squat requires flexibility in the calves and Achilles tendons, many beginners struggle to squat below 45-degrees. To overcome this use two-inch spacers to raise your heels.

- If you haven't attempted an overhead squat before, it is wise to practice with an unloaded bar or broomstick. The following teaching points apply to trainers using a light bar.
- Hold the bar at your front and space your hands wide; the bar should be level with your hips.
- If you're using spacers, it's best to manoeuvre your heels on them before getting the bar into position.
- Organise your feet so that they are just over shoulder-width apart.
- Raise the bar above your head ensuing to apply tension by pulling it apart as though you are tearing it in two.
- Keeping the bar directly above your head, under control squat down to 90-degrees.
- Pause momentarily before returning to the start position.

General advice

- Ensure that you can safely perform all the exercises before undertaking the workout. I only mention this because the overhead squat is quite complex and requires considerable practice before anywhere close to competency is achieved.

- To those who plan to step in the ring with the 10-ton challenge, it's wise to draw up a set/rep tally chart before pulling on your gloves. By implementing this advice you'll easily and accurately be able to track progress.
- Another point of note for the 10-ton competitors. The number of sets and reps represented in the trackers have been calculated against the weights in parenthesis following each exercise. If you plan to change the weight ($\pm$), you will of course need to recalibrate those reps so that you achieve a combined lift of 2500kg.
- *To account for those extra goblet squat reps. Five sets of 15 reps of a 32kg KB equates to 2400kg lifted. Thus, we're left with a debt of 100kg. No matter, that's easily remunerated. Four additional swings are all that's need to balance the books. (To pre-empt those pedantic types, yes, I concede, 19 reps put you in credit by 28kg. But better to have a surfeit than a deficit, wouldn't you agree?)

What is functional fitness?

Functional fitness consists of a mix of strength, power, muscular endurance, and cardio. The person who possesses functional fitness will routinely participate in a wide range of training modalities.

Another characteristic of functional fitness is the ability to transition through different training methods with relative ease. For example, a functionally fit individual would have no problem completing a barbell complex (Workout 19) after a gruelling set of hill sprints (Workout 8).

Why is functional fitness important?

The pursuit of functional fitness is important for a whole host of reasons. However, instead of boring you with a long list, I'll briefly outline what I consider to be the two primary reasons why you should consider cultivating this coveted physical competency.

First, because functional training incorporates a wide range of exercise methodologies, it develops strength, muscle endurance and cardiovascular fitness. Consequently, by pursuing functional fitness, you will become a more well-rounded trainer.

Second, the physical functionality that this training approach promotes is more reflective of day-to-day tasks. As I've argued elsewhere, rare is it that we are required to execute a strict triceps extension, or a slow lateral raise capped with a two-second 'peak contraction' *squeeze!*

Typically, daily tasks such as DIY, gardening, and household chores involve the whole body. Functional fitness training, which includes performing dynamic exercises like the kettlebell thruster and powerbag deadlift, is representative of the physical requirements of everyday life.

The benefits of functional fitness training
- ✓ Improves whole-body fitness
- ✓ Rectifies fitness imbalances
- ✓ Can make everyday tasks easier
- ✓ Facilitates positive changes in body composition
- ✓ Enhances muscular definition
- ✓ Develops the main components of fitness

How to train for functional fitness

Training for functional fitness is easier than you might think. In fact, if you exercise regularly, chances are you already participate in some form of functional fitness.

To modify a pre-existing exercise regime to one that includes functional elements often only requires a few minor adaptations. For example, if you currently train in a conventional manner – sets and reps weightlifting – by making a couple of alterations to your workout you could be on the fast track to functional fitness.

One simple way of training functionally is to make a circuit out of your static workout.

Circuit training
I argued in the introduction that circuit training is a superior form of training and one that promotes complete physical competency. Well, it's also one of the most effective exercise methodologies for improving functional fitness. As we've previously discussed, to develop physical functionality you must train the main components of fitness equally. This is difficult to do if you primarily focus on one exercise method such as resistance or cardio.

Because circuit training combines multiple exercise methods, it naturally promotes functional fitness. In a single circuit, you could include strength, muscular endurance, and cardio exercises. Thus, in one workout, almost the entire training spectrum will be covered.

CrossFit is the ultimate in functional training
Following on from above, CrossFit (which is kind of like circuit training on steroids) is one of the purest forms of functional fitness training. CrossFit athletes are the quintessential Jack of all fitness trainers.

It's not enough for a CrossFitter to specialise in any one fitness component. The consummate CrossFit athlete must develop all aspects of their fitness in relatively equal measures.

Throughout the CrossFit games, competitors could be required to complete maximal Olympic lifts, row a marathon, conquer a calisthenics complex, and even tackle strongman-style events.

To stand any chance of surviving, let alone amassing enough points to get within a muscle-up of the podium, CrossFit athletes must forge complete functional fitness.

Functional fitness training plan
If you're desirous of developing functional fitness the following plan can help. The plan has been designed to provide you with a simplified framework of how you could structure a training routine that promotes functional fitness.

You can either implement the plan as it is or tailor it to suit your exercise preferences and current training commitment. Alternatively, instead of implementing the plan proper, you can have a go at the individual training sessions that feature throughout. By opting for this approach, you'll get a flavour for this style of training, which will enable you ascertain if it is palatable, and you will be provided with weeks of workouts.

You'll notice that the plan has been organised into three levels: beginner, intermediate, and advanced. This has been done to make it more accessible to a wider audience.

How to use the functional fitness plan

- Select the level most appropriate to your current level of fitness
- Structure the workouts across your training week
- Ensure to complete a progressive 10-minute warm-up prior to every workout
- Conclude each workout with a cool-down and stretch

	Functional Fitness Plan		
	Beginner	**Intermediate**	**Advanced**
Monday	2000-metre row Dumbbell-body weight complex: Barbell thruster 10 reps Press-ups 10 reps Farmer's walk 10-metres Burpees 10 reps Single-arm dumbbell snatch 5 reps Plank 10-seconds Squat jumps 10 reps Repeat the complex as many times as possible in 10-minutes	2000-metre row Dumbbell-body weight complex: Barbell thruster 10 reps Press-ups 10 reps Farmer's walk 10-metres Burpees 10 reps Single-arm dumbbell snatch 5 reps Plank 10-seconds Squat jumps 10 reps Repeat the complex as many times as possible in 20-minutes	2000-metre row Dumbbell-body weight complex: Barbell thruster 10 reps Press-ups 10 reps Farmer's walk 10-metres Burpees 10 reps Single-arm dumbbell snatch 5 reps Plank 10-seconds Squat jumps 10 reps Repeat the complex as many times as possible in 30-minutes
Tuesday			3k run 10 X 100-metre hill sprints

			Kettlebell / Calisthenics AMRAP:
			3-min KB swings 1-min rest 3-min Burpees 1-min rest 3-min KB squats 1-min rest 3-min Press-ups 1-min rest 3-min KB clean 1-min rest 3-min Burpees
	Rest day	Rest Day	
			Objective: amass as many reps as possible in 3-minutes
Wednesday	2k run 10 X 50-metre hill sprints Kettlebell / Calisthenics AMRAP: 2-min KB swings 1-min rest 2-min Burpees 1-min rest 2-min KB squats 1-min rest 2-min Press-ups 1-min rest 2-min KB clean 1-min rest 2-min Burpees	2k run 10 X 100-metre hill sprints Kettlebell / Calisthenics AMRAP: 3-min KB swings 1-min rest 3-min Burpees 1-min rest 3-min KB squats 1-min rest 3-min Press-ups 1-min rest 3-min KB clean 1-min rest 3-min Burpees	2000-metre row Barbell complex: Deadlift 10 reps Bent-over row 10 reps Hang cleans 10 reps Front squats 10 reps Standing shoulder press 10 reps Repeat the complex as many times as possible in 30-minutes 2000-metre row: maintain a high pace

	Objective: amass as many reps as possible in 3-minutes	Objective: amass as many reps as possible in 3-minutes	
Thursday	Rest day	2000-metre row Barbell complex: Deadlift 10 reps Bent-over row 10 reps Hang cleans 10 reps Front squats 10 reps Standing shoulder press 10 reps Repeat the complex as many times as possible in 20-minutes. 1000-metre row: maintain a high pace	4- to 6-mile slow run (or equivalent distance/time cardio exercise)
Friday	2000-metre row Barbell complex: Deadlift 10 reps Bent-over row 10 reps Hang cleans 10 reps Front squats 10 reps Standing shoulder press 10 reps Repeat the complex as many times as possible in 10-minutes	2000-metre row 3 X 5-minute AMRAP Barbell thruster (light weight) Kettlebell swing Farmer's walk (metres in 5-minutes) 2000-metre run or airdyne bike: maintain a high pace	2000-metre row 4 X 5-minute AMRAP Barbell thruster (light weight) Kettlebell swing Farmer's walk (metres in 5-minutes) Deadlift 3000-metre run or airdyne bike: maintain a high pace

Saturday	Rest day	4- to 6-mile slow run (or equivalent distance/time cardio exercise)	4- to 6-mile slow run (or equivalent distance/time cardio exercise)
Sunday	Observe the Sabbath	Observe the Sabbath	Observe the Sabbath

Workout 48
Train Hard Fight Easy

If you work hard in training, the fight is easy.
– Manny Pacquiao – eight-division world champion

The health and fitness benefits of boxing have long been understood. Few sports or exercise disciplines incorporate such a broad range of fitness components as does the sweet art of pugilism.

In a typical boxing session, the pugilist will need to demonstrate superior cardiovascular resolve and muscular endurance output. Moreover, the boxer must maintain mental focus as they coordinate their body through a series of complex and explosive movements.

And this is just training! We haven't considered combat yet.

But that is one of the most common misunderstandings of boxing – viz. that in order participate in boxing you have to fight. This, of course, is not even nearly true. You can still reap the many benefits the sport has to offer without throwing a single aggressive punch. And the list of benefits is impressive. They include:

✓ Fat burning
✓ Enhanced muscle tonality
✓ Improved bone density
✓ Increased cardio-respiratory performance
✓ Augmented muscular endurance
✓ Improved core stability
✓ Increased power

✓ Enhanced reaction time and coordination *and* agility

✓ Develop a combat skill

✓ Stress relief

You want some of these benefits? Then read on . . .

How it works

Nothing fancy. No glitz or glamour . . . just a run-of-the-mill, spit 'n sawdust boxing workout. But, and at heart we all know *this* to be true, the old school training methods are the best.

So how does it work?

Warm-up well. Set a three-minute repeat countdown timer with a minute rest. Work through the three main phases of a boxing workout: shadow boxing, bag/pad training, calisthenics.

Concluding the main workout, cool-down, stretch off, and then hit the showers.

Key points

- Warm-up!
- Using a countdown timer, set an interval split of three-minutes to one-minute.
- For three-minutes maintain a high work rate ensuring to stay active until the bell.
- Take your minute rest but be ready to go the moment the next round starts.
- Conclude your workout with a cool-down and stretch.

Workout

Phase 1: 10-minute warm-up – for the first couple of minutes perform a series of mobility exercises. Rotate the shoulders, hips and ankles. Also, complete several controlled jumps. This will prepare the calves and tendons of the feet for skipping.

Now for the remaining 8-minutes skip. Start off slow building the tempo as the time elapses.

Phase 2: 2 X 3-minute rounds of shadow boxing (1-minute rest) – preferably in front of a mirror practice your pugilism. Focus on throwing controlled punches and concentrate on the quality of your technique. The tempo or intensity should be high enough so that you keep the warmth generated during the warm-up.

Phase 3: 10 X 3-minute rounds of bag work (1-minute rest) – once you've wrapped your hands properly, gloved up and set a timer, work the bag ensuring, again, to focus on technique and the execution of your punches. Remember, you shouldn't mindlessly wail away on the punch bag like a Saturday night drunkard thinking he's Muhammad Ali. Yes, your work ethic should be high, and you should be sweating profusely. But you should still remain in control of your pugilism – that is, maintain a defensive guard and face your (imaginary) opponent at all times.

Phase 4: 10-minute conditioning calisthenics AMRAP – for ten continuous minutes you are to work through the following exercises performing ten repetitions on each before moving on:

- Press-ups
- Burpees
- Plank (10-second count)
- Hill climbers*
- Squat jumps

Phase 5: 2 X 3-minute rounds of shadow boxing (1-minute rest) – preferably in front of a mirror practice your pugilism. Focus on throwing controlled punches and concentrate on the quality of your technique. The tempo or intensity should be relaxed; this is the cool-down phase.

Phase 6: 5-minute whole-body stretch – see the 10-minute stretching plan below.

General advice

- *What's a *hill climber* when it's at home? The humble hill climber is a variation of the squat thrust. The slight difference being, instead of pumping both feet out and back together, as you would with a squat thrust, the legs are pumped alternatively – somewhat like a pair of pistons. Still confused? Google it!

- Why don't you do something out of the ordinary and go join a local boxing club? Even if it's just for one training session. I'm being serious. For the tuppence it'll cost you to gain admittance, you'll likely receive the best workout of your life. And you never know, you might even enjoy it.

- *But what if I don't have a boxing bag and gloves?* (And what if you're too much of a wuss to join a local boxing club?) Do what the legendary amateur boxer Felix Savon did and fill an old sack with sand and rock and get your mum to make you mitts from discarded hessian. Sling the sack from a tree, glove up, and start smacking away. What's your excuse?

Workout 49
Five More EMOMs

As the saying goes, you can never have too much of a good thing. Because I'm a big believer in that sagacious maxim, certainly when applied to fitness training, I invite you to test the mettle of your physicality over the anvil of the following five EMOM workouts.

The EMOMs below are comprised of an eclectic mix of exercises. From Girevoy Sports-style kettlebell cycles to CrossFit-inspired barbell complexes, there's an EMOM here for any and all fitness fetishes.

But if you're scratching your noggin over how EMOMs work, flick forward to Appendix A, Circuit Design, where you'll find a comprehensive overview.

Key points

- A general warm-up suggestion suitable for all proceeding workouts has been provided.
- A 'How it works' explanation is situated beneath each EMOM.

Warm-up

Prior to participating in the EMOM workouts, ensure to complete a 10-minute warm-up. The warm-up should include a cardiovascular element – such as rowing, the cross-trainer, or skipping. Also, to prepare the muscles for resistance training, sprinkle the warm-up with a few low-intensity sets of the exercises that feature in the EMOM.

Workouts

EMOM 1: 20-minute kettlebell single-arm clean to press cycle

Minute 1 to 5: 4 reps each arm
Minute 6 to 10: 6 reps each arm
Minute 11 to 15: 8 reps each arm
Minute 16 to 20: 10 reps each arm

There's no denying it, that final five-minutes is going to induce a nasty burn both in the lungs and deltoids. Also, you'll be left with very little rest between sets. But it's always best, I believe, to conclude your EMOM with a bang.

You can approach this session in two different ways. The first: complete all the reps on one arm before changing. The second: change arms on the conclusion of each rep.

Personally, I prefer the second approach. However, when changing between each successive rep, one tends to incur a minor time penalty as you are forced to linger for a split second at the lowest position to swop hands. This won't be a problem from minute one through to minute 10. But when you hit those big rep sets it's going to eat into your rest.

EMOM 2: 12-minute alternate dumbbell thruster to double unders . . . x 2!

Minute 1: 10 reps dumbbell thruster
Minute 2: 20 double unders

Repeat until you conclude minute 12, 20 double unders. Before initiating the second set of 12-minutes, complete 2000m on the ergo rower. This isn't supposed to be a rest by the way. Your row pace should remain competitive. (Note: if you can't do double unders then skip as fast as physically possible. If you can't skip at all, either teach yourself and come back when you can or sprint on the spot.)

This EMOM is a near-perfect unification of resistance and cardio. Consequently, it is pretty much a complete session. Dumbbell thrusters – superior to their barbell kin – stimulate about 90% of our musculature. Skipping, if not the best form of cardio exercise, is certainly situated somewhere at the top (supposing a hierarchy of cardio superiority). Combined, these two exercises make for a fabulous fitness friendship.

EMOM 3: 5/10/15/20/25 or 30-minute whole-body strength

Minute 1: 6 reps military press
Minute 2: 6 reps bench press
Minute 3: 6 reps bent-over rows
Minute 4: 6 reps deadlifts
Minute 5: 6 reps squat

First, before starting this session, you need to determine suitable weights for each exercise. You could always make life easy for yourself and settle for a percentage of your overall body weight – 50%, 60%, 70%, etc. However, the only drawback with this approach is that for certain exercises – deadlifts and squats – your strength won't be adequately tested. I'll leave this conundrum for you to ponder.

The way I approached this session is by using an Olympic barbell loaded with two 20kg bumper plates. I didn't stop the clock until I'd completed six continuous cycles. I stick to 60kg because a) it more than adequately challenges my physicality across the range of exercises listed above; b) I like to use the same bar because to get it in position for the military press and squats, I am required to complete a full clean and press, which compounds the strenuousness of the session; and c) I can't be doing with faffing over changing up and down weights.

EMOM 4: 3/6/9/12/15/18/21/24/27 or 30-minute clean and press pyramid

Minute 1: 6 reps deadlifts
Minute 2: 6 reps hang-cleans

Minute 3: 6 push press

The perceptive reader, or CrossFit/Olympic lifting enthusiast, will notice that the three individual exercises that form this EMOM, when pieced together, comprise the clean and jerk. By breaking down a complex movement we are afforded the opportunity to perfect (or improve) each individual phase while also enjoying an excellent workout in the process.

Variations of this system abound. For example, you could cut the reps right back and complete two or three reps of each isolated phase in the same minute. Or you could perform, say, two deadlifts into two hang cleans into two push presses. Rest, then repeat for the desired number of minutes.

EMOM 5: 24-minutes of pure calisthenics

Minute 1: 20 reps press-ups
Minute 2: 6 reps pull-ups
Minute 3: 10 reps full-weight dips
Minute 4: 10 hanging leg raises
Minute 5: 10 reps burpees
Minute 6: 100-metres sprint
Repeat four more times.

This EMOM, basic though it be, has got a military flavour to it. But that's not a bad thing. After all, the military produces some superbly fit people. Also, what this session will show you, if you decide to have a bash, is that you really don't need much equipment or a fancy gym to keep in shape. Those five exercises will work every inch of your physicality. Seriously, no myofibril will be left unmolested – for good or bad.

Now, depending on the current capacity of your muscular endurance, you might either want to decrease or increase the rep ranges assigned to each exercise.

In my experience, many trainers struggle to perform pull-ups. Basically, few people possess the requisite strength to heave their corporal mass through a full concentric contraction of the arms.

If you are not yet strong enough to execute a pull-up, don't fret! Simply change the exercise or, if you can find a bar about waist height, do inverted or modified pull-ups instead.

General advice

- When EMOMing life is made so much easier if you use a repeat countdown timer. Manually resetting the timer is a recipe for EMOM procrastination. Also, it adversely impacts the rhythm of the workout.
- Don't be afraid to modify or amend the workouts to suit your current physical capacity. If the reps are too high (or too low), change them! If the prescribed number of minutes is too numerous, knock 'em down a bit!

Workout 50
The Grand Finale: Marathon Row

The marathon is the White Whale among rowing enthusiasts and fitness sadists. To complete the distance in a single stint is a significant physical feat. But the social kudos it confers and bragging rights it bequeaths makes this monumental undertaking worth the hours of suffering.

After all, how many people can say that they've rowed a marathon?

Before attempting this gruelling challenge, you will need to invest in preparatory training. As the saying goes, prior preparation prevents poor performance. But how much training you do will largely be dictated by your objective going into the marathon – are you happy to complete the distance or are you desirous of a specific time?

For example, if you harbour the ambition of covering the distance in a single sitting, then a month or two might afford the requisite training time to achieve this modest outcome.

However, this of course does depend on your current level of fitness and how much rowing experience you have. If you are untrained, rarely participate in aerobic exercise, or have recently started a training programme, you may need to spend upwards of six-months preparing.

If you are well trained and row regularly, then you may well be ready for the challenge after a week or two of training. But if you set your sights on a specific time, say under three-hours (2:05/500m), you would be wise to implement a training programme.

But why row a marathon?

Besides the fact that completing such a monumental physical challenge is a significant achievement, and one to be proud of, preparing for the marathon will provide you with months of training focus.

Having worked as an exercise professional for many years, I've noticed that one of the most common hurdles people struggle to overcome is the lack of training motivation.

For some people, if there is no end objective to their training, if they're not working towards a specific goal, they quickly lose motivation. A lack of motivation leads to inconsistent training participation and, in far too many cases, the person quitting exercise all together.

Resolving to complete a marathon will provide you with a training purpose while also bringing structure to your exercise routine. In addition, rowing is arguably one of the best single exercises for improving body composition and developing aerobic fitness.

As well as improving cardio-respiratory performance, rowing also builds stamina and strength in the two major muscle groups – those of the back and legs. Few other cardiovascular exercises develop whole-body fitness as effectively as rowing.

How I prepared for the marathon row

I'll be honest, I didn't implement or undertake anything that would even remotely qualify as a programme. I'd been hankering after the marathon for months (ever since I saw CrossFit athletes complete the distance in the 2019 games). Problem is, I'm very unscientific in my training approach. However, I happened upon an idea.

As part of the **Hungry4Fitness** 'Week in The Life' series, where I attempt to survive the training regime of a professional athlete, I decided to have a bash at the training programme of an Olympic rower.

So, a week prior to attempting the marathon, I implemented the training programme of an Olympic rower, which saw me cover 170,000-metres in six days. This provided the preparatory groundwork for the gruelling challenge.

I'm not suggesting that you try this strategy. As it is a bad strategy. But what it's supposed to illustrate is that, even with just a week of solid training (I was averaging 25,000-metres per day), it is possible to prepare the requisite physicality to complete the marathon distance.

Going into the marathon I set my sights on an average pace of 1:59/500. However, after 30,000-metres, my cardio deserted me, and I limped to the finish line having sustained a pace of 2:03/500. That was annoying because, if I'd prepared properly, as I'm advising you to do, I may well have achieved my goal. Learn from my mistake, make sure you prepare.

Though the marathon row is, by anyone's standards, an imposing test of fitness and mental toughness, you could complete the distance with the correct training commitment. To support you in this arduous undertaking, I have included a generic rowing programme and a list of top tips.

If implemented and followed, the programme can help lay the requisite cardiovascular foundations required to make the crossing without foundering on the rocks of fatigue. The list of tips provides methods and strategies to attenuate the inevitable discomfort and suffering that all marathon rowers encounter. Of course, it's unrealistic to expect to avoid physical adversity when engaging in sustained activity for protracted periods. However, while the hurt cannot be completely obviated, it can be softened and smoothed somewhat.

How to prepare for a marathon row

Below you will discover a blueprint of a four-month training programme. The programme is supposed to provide you with an outline of how you might prepare to row 42.195 consecutive metres – aka a marathon.

Because the programme is generalised it would be inadvisable to follow it exactly. Use it as a framework around which to construct a more comprehensive and tailored programme.

T-minus four months – preparing the fitness groundwork

Over a four-month period prior to embarking on the marathon challenge, aim to complete ten 10,000-metre rows. This will see you cover 10,000m every week for four months. By following this simple training method, you will progressively develop the physical capacity to sustain substantial row stints.

Of course, in addition to the weekly 10,000-metre mini-marathons, you will also be completing shorter distances.

T-minus two months – build up

At T-minus two months you will start to increase the intensity of your pre-marathon rowing training. Over a four-week period, aim to complete four one-hour and two 20,000-metre rows.

It is best to space these row sessions across the month as evenly as possible. You might decide to complete the one-hour rows midweek and the big 20,000-metre distances on the weekend. By following a logical methodology, you will have more time to rest and recover after each row.

The objective for these lengthy stints is to maintain a methodical pace at or near the pace you plan to sustain for the marathon. In addition to enhancing fitness and building self-confidence, you are also developing an understanding of your physical capabilities. Furthermore, extensive row distances enable you to assess how your body holds up and whether your stroke or seating position need adjusting.

If you start too fast and tire – or worse over exhaust yourself – this could result in poor performance or failure to finish. These outcomes will adversely impact your psychology going into the competition.

T-minus 12 days – trial run

At the 12-day point attempt a 30,000-metre row. Completing a distance close to that of the competition will afford you the opportunity to assess how your body and mind respond. If they (you) respond well, and you conclude the 30,000-metres feeling as though you could have gone on for a further 12,195, this is telling you that you are ready.

Furthermore, the 30,000-metres will also provide you with an insight into any issues that need addressing prior to undertaking the marathon. For example, it will enable you to answer the following questions:

- Is my position on the rower comfortable and do I need extra seat padding?
- Is one water bottle enough or will I need two?
- Were those energy snacks beneficial?
- Is my pacing objective too ambitious?
- Will I need to enforce reduced pacing or short walk periods?

Day 0 – Marathon row

On the day all you can do is prepare. Perhaps consider putting together a checklist of items you think you might need to see you through the distance. Procure the items and, prior to undertaking the marathon, prepare your environment.

If you are completing the distance on a gym rower, it is prudent to check that the batteries in the Pm monitor have plenty of charge. Also, you might want to move kit around to create a bit more space.

Before disembarking make sure that all your provisions – water, nutrition, towel – are within reach. When everything is in place, psych yourself up and go for it.

Remember this last point, it's a marathon, not a sprint – so don't start off too fast. Take your time, ease into the rhythm, remain faithful to your strategy, and resist the temptation to deviate from your target pace.

Hungry4Fitness
Marathon Row Training Programme

Time stages	Training Process
Four months out	**Basic Groundwork** Complete at least ten 10,000-metre rows over two months. In addition, work through twenty 5,000 and 2,500-metre rows.
Two months out	**Build Up** Over four weeks, complete four one-hour pieces, and then complete two 20,000-meter pieces. Use interval or repetition format: ➢ Divide 60-minutes by going at a moderate pace for 2:30, then going easy for 30-seconds. Repeat. ➢ Divide 20,000m by completing 500m @22spm*, 300m @24spm, and 200m @26spm. Repeat 20 times. When you are not doing one of the longer distances, continue training with 30- to 45-minute rows. *spm = strokes per minute
12 days out	**Trial Run** Complete one 30,000-metre row. See how your body holds up and take this opportunity to address any issues. Test out the nutritional provisions that you plan to consume on the day.
Marathon!	**Challenge Day** Prior to embarking on the marathon enjoy a pre-challenge rest day. Also, ensure that you are adequately fed and watered. It is advisable to spend a bit of time before the event preparing your provisions: seat padding, nutrition, hydration.

> Don't forget, just do your best, don't put any unnecessary
> pressure on yourself, and enjoy the experience.

Timing and pace

- Typically, marathons take around three to four hours to complete. By maintaining an average pace of 2:05/500m, you'll achieve a time of just less than three hours.
- On the day of the challenge, nerves will be high, and you'll be anxious to get stuck in. This is completely natural. However, resist starting out too hard and stick to your pace plan. In fact, it's best to start off under pace and build up over the first 5,000-metres.

Tips for success

- Hydrate! Hydrate! Hydrate!
- Rest when your body needs it.
- On the build-up to the challenge increase the amount of rest between training sessions by varying when you work out each day.
- Consider monitoring your heart rate at rest during your pre-marathon training.
- Know how to be comfortable on the indoor rower.
- Work on improving – nay *perfecting* – your rowing technique.
- Make sure you have fresh batteries in your Pm monitor because the last thing you want is it cutting out on the final metre!
- Gloves can reduce blisters and sore spots; however, you should test them out before attempting the marathon: bulky training gloves can induce fatigue in the forearms.
- It is advisable to have water, snacks, towels, and tissues to hand during your attempt.
- There's no shame in taking short breaks throughout the distance. Every 10,000-metres, say, you could dismount the rower, take a short walk and carry on (**remember**, though, the Performance Monitor shuts down after a couple of

minutes of inactivity). Alternatively, you could periodically reduce the pace for 1000-metres. Once you've recovered work back to pace until the next rest. So, keep your breaks short or keep pressing **Change Display** or **Display** to keep the monitor on.

- Finally, good luck!

Congratulations!

You've Completed the

Hungry4Fitness *Book of Circuits*

Volume 2.

Appendix A
Circuit & Workout Design

Below I have briefly outlined a range of classic and contemporary circuit and workout designs. They can be used as guides to help you understand the circuits throughout this book or as templates that you can use to create your own workouts.

Circular circuit

The circular circuit is by far the oldest and most straightforward design. After establishing the exercise stations and deciding on the method of approach – specific rep range or time duration – you would start at the first exercise and proceed to complete one lap. The objective is to complete either a pre-specified number of laps or as many laps as possible in a given time. Adequate circuit durations range from 10-minutes to one hour.

Stations

The number of individual stations the circuit contains is entirely up to you the designer. However, in saying that, I would suggest a lower limit of no fewer than six and an upper maximum of no more than 20.

If our circular circuit contains only a small number of exercises, we will inevitably progress through the stations too quickly which can impact muscle recovery. Consequently, we are more likely to fatigue early which will impede momentum.

But, on the other side of the extreme, if we over-populate the circuit with stations, it will take too long to complete a lap which defeats the object this design. Thus, the number of stations must be just right. To keep things simple, stick to a station range of between eight and 12.

Exercises

There is no right or wrong exercise choice for a circuit. In saying that, though, it does make sense to select exercises that confer a desired fitness benefit. For example, if you wanted to develop strength in all the major muscle groups, you might populate your circuit with compound exercises. In addition, the ordering of the exercises could follow a logical sequence starting with either the lower body or upper body muscle groups. As you progressed through the circuit each muscle group would be worked in turn.

However, that's merely an idea and, of course, you do not have to follow such a prescriptive design. You can throw off the straitjacket of convention and go so far as to select exercises at random. If you were organising a circular circuit for a group, after deciding on the number of stations, you could scribble exercises on pieces of paper, scrunch them up, toss them into a hat, and get the group members to decide the design fate of the circuit. (For kicks and giggles, write 100 burpees on all the pieces of paper. Love it!)

Concerning the fitness component that exercises engage, it is perfectly acceptable to mix strength with muscular endurance movements. Also, there is absolutely no harm whatsoever including cardio and calisthenics exercises in the same circuit. In fact, such a circuit is far more reflective of the physical demands of daily life.

Repetitions/time

Now that we've covered the mechanics of the circular circuit, let's consider the method of approach. We have the option of applying a specific repetition range – say 10 reps per exercise – or a time duration – such as 20-seconds – at each station.

Deciding between time and repetitions is of course personal preference. However, in my experience, when conducting a group circuit, you should always stick with time due to the inevitability of participants completing their reps before others. The last thing we want in a group circuit is participants standing around waiting for others to finish. Fixed time durations prevent this from happening.

When applying time or repetitions you may want to consider applying an incremental ascending ordering. For example, if you decided on timed stations, you could begin with 30-seconds per station and incrementally increase it by 10-, 20- or 30-seconds after each completed lap. Adopting this method progressively raises the intensity and training volume over the course of the session. Typically, the final lap of a circular circuit is the most physically demanding – when the end is in sight.

Rest/recovery

The conventional way a circular circuit would operate is after completion of every full lap a short rest is taken. Usually for the rest period the participants would walk a couple of laps around the circuit/gym hall (depending on space of course). Active recovery is far more beneficial than sitting down or standing still. It can be a lot harder to get the body going again once you have stopped.

Optimally, rest periods should not exceed 1-minute 30-seconds. But this depends on the fitness levels of the participants. A group comprised of untrained people may require the scheduling of longer rest periods. Doubling or even tripling the above recommended rest time will enable untrained participants to complete the circuit. This not only ensures that they enjoy the many fitness benefits circuit training confers but will also bolster self-efficacy. Being forced to quit a circuit in the presence of peers and contemporaries is both humiliating and confidence-destroying. Adequate recovery can mitigate this demoralising outcome.

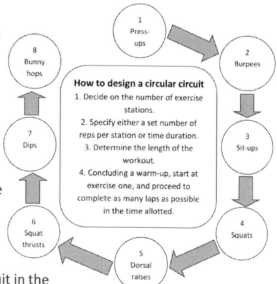

In contrast, intermediate and advanced trainers might decide to take only a 30-second rest or abolish it altogether.

The best tactic here is to experiment with a varied range of rest durations. However, we must remember that the intensity of a circuit should remain high. If the rest period is extensive the circuit will ultimately denigrate into just another gym session thus losing its primary function.

Circular circuit overview

- The optimal number of exercises that a circular circuit should feature consists of between eight and 12.
- Either a time duration or repetition count can be applied to the exercises.
- It is good practice to structure the time/rep range in ascending incremental ordering. For example, lap one 30-seconds, lap two 45-seconds, lap three 60-seconds, lap four 90-seocnds, and the final lap 120-seconds. The same method can just as easily be applied when opting for repetitions. For example, lap one 10 reps, lap two 20 reps, lap three 30 reps, and so on. However, for the reasons outlined above, applying reps for group circuits is inadvisable.
- Typically, a circular circuit will span the duration of 45-minutes. This does not include the warm-up, cool-down, and stretch phases.
- Any exercise could be included within the circuit.
- It matters not a jot how the exercises are ordered – pull them out of a hat if the fancy takes.
- The rest period length is dictated ultimately by the fitness levels of the participants. Ideally, recovery should not exceed 10 per cent of the time it takes to complete one lap.

Lineal circuit

The lineal circuit is by far my favourite design for the fact that psychologically it seems to finish a lot quicker than the other formats. When embarking on a lineal circuit it's rather like making a journey. Because there is a definite start and end point progress is salient, which is both rewarding and motivational.

A circular circuit, in contrast, can sometimes make you feel as though you are stuck in a never-ending loop. If the stations are populated with bland body weight exercises, this can make for a monotonous training experience. Thus, to add a bit of colour to a circular circuit, the architect must apply their creative license when selecting exercises.

This design demand is not as acutely felt when building a lineal circuit. Whereas the same exercise might be performed again and again over the course of the circular circuit, this is not the case with the lineal design. Once the exercise has been completed you move on to the next along the line. Think of the lineal circuit as a training to-do list.

As illustrated in the diagram below, starting at the first exercise, which in Example 1 is press-ups, you would complete the prescribed number of reps. On concluding the final rep of the first exercise, put a cross through it then proceed to the next in line. Carry on in this fashion until every exercise on your training to-do list has been crossed off.

To make the circuit run smoother ensure you have it written on a sheet of paper. Ticking off the exercises as you go helps keep track of progress while also providing a motivational stimulus.

Example 1	Example 2	Example 3
1. Press-ups – 50r	1. Rower – 500m	1. Squat – 50r (30kg)
2. Burpees – 25r	2. Bike – 2k	2. Deadlift – 50r (50kg)
3. Sit-ups – 100r	3. Running – 1000m	3. Cleans – 50r (40kg)
4. Etc.	4. Etc.	4. Ad infinitum

Exercises

Because each station in a lineal circuit is visited only once the number of exercises and repetitions is typically greater. It is also for this reason why they contain considerably more stations. I've organised lineal circuits in the past that were comprised of 30 exercises.

When deciding on how many exercises and reps you are going to use, make sure that you are aware of your limitations first. Believe me when I say it is very easy to get carried away adding exercises and reps/distances. And what takes a second and a smear of ink can cost minutes and many drops of sweat.

Rest/recovery

We should not rest during a lineal circuit. The objective is to complete all the exercises in the shortest time possible.

Kilogram/repetition circuit

Some years ago, I wanted to set a world record for lifting one-million kilograms in 15-hours. Unfortunately, the organisation that I approached to oversee the challenge dismissed it on account of the multitude of similar records. While batting back and forth correspondence, I put in some hefty training sessions in preparation for if I got the green light. One such session saw me lift a combined weight of 250,000 kilograms in two and a half hours. Even though I never got the chance to put this hard work into practice, it was nevertheless brilliant training.

The circuit that I had devised for the challenge was a ten-station circular circuit. One full lap equated to 10,000 kilograms of weight lifted. For challenges such as this it is best to use a light resistance – I was using a 25kg barbell. These sessions are easy to design, and they confer many fitness benefits such as burning fat, increasing muscular endurance, and improving muscle definition.

The basic principle of how the kilogram challenge works is as follows. A single bicep curl of a 20kg barbell equates to a combined total lift of 20kgs. Nothing too complicated there. Now, if you curled the same barbell a second time that would double your total taking it up to 40 kilograms. Completing a set of 100 repetitions on a 20kg barbell equates to 2,000 kilograms lifted. As you've by now no doubt realised, all we are doing is multiplying the weight by the repetitions. It is quite surprising how much weight can be shifted in an hour's session. However, unlike the circular and lineal circuits, when it comes to accumulating kilograms the ordering of exercises and the weight selected require consideration.

Prior to picking up a weight, it is important to spend some time considering how the exercises are going to be ordered. Arbitrarily pairing exercises could hinder the fluidity of the session and greatly reduce the overall weight lifted. It is advisable to avoid pairing exercises that engage the same muscle groups.

Combining exercises that activate different muscles, such as pairing bench press with bent-over row (chest and back), or deadlift with squats (back and legs), allows one muscle group to recover while the other is working. This enables the trainer to oscillate back and forth between exercises without resting. In my experience, this is by the most efficient means of maximising the number of kilograms that can be lifted throughout the circuit. In the following table I have compiled a list of optimal and suboptimal muscle group pairings.

Muscle Group Pairings	
Optimal Pairings	**Suboptimal Pairings**
Biceps + Triceps Chest + Biceps Back + Chest Back + Triceps Shoulders + Back Legs + any of the above Abdominals + any of the above	Back + Biceps Chest + Triceps Shoulders + Chest Triceps + Shoulders

The three main points to take into consideration when designing a kilogram accumulation circuit include:

1. Pairing of muscle groups
2. Organisation of exercises
3. Resistance ranges

Before commencing a kilogram circuit, I will calculate how many reps and how much weight is required to meet a specific target. For example, I will select two exercises that work different muscle groups with a goal of reaching, say, 2,500kg each. A barbell weight of 25kg lifted 100 times will meet this target. These reps will not be performed in one set but split into manageable chunks – usually sets of 25 reps.

Exercises and weight	Repetitions					Total lifted
Bench press – 25kg	~~20r~~	~~20r~~	~~20r~~	20r	20r	2,500kg
Bent-over row – 25kg	~~20r~~	~~20r~~	20r	20r	20r	2,500kg

As exemplified in the diagram above, you would transition from bench press to bent-over row nonstop until all boxes are crossed off. Setting aside a few minutes to create a tracker like this one, crude though it is, can help make the session flow a lot smoother. When you are tired and sweaty the last thing you want to be doing is jotting down reps and tallying up weights.

Of course, there is always the option of doing the calculations when you get home. However, having it written out as displayed in the example above, not only makes life that bit easier but also acts as a powerful motivational tool. Hopefully you agree. If you don't, before dismissing my method give it a whirl and see how you get on.

Arnold Schwarzenegger outlines a similar motivational tactic in his magnum opus *The Encyclopaedia of Modern Bodybuilding*. Discussing his idiosyncratic style of monitoring reps and boosting training motivation, Schwarzenegger tells us that

'When I began to train, I wrote everything down – training routines, sets and reps, diet, everything. And I kept this up right through my 1980 Mr. Olympia victory. I would come into the gym and draw out a line on the wall in chalk for every set I intended to do. I would always to five sets of each movement. So for example, the marks ////////// on my chest day would stand for five sets of Bench Press and five sets of Dumbbell Flys. I would reach up and cross each line as I did the set. So when I finished Benches the marks would look like X X X X X /////, and I would never think to myself, Should I do three sets today, or four? I always knew it was five and just went ahead and did them. Watching those marks march across the wall as I did my workout gave me a tremendous sense of satisfaction and accomplishment. They were like an invading army crushing all opposition in its path. This visual feedback helped me to keep my training goals clearly in mind, and reinforced my determination to push myself to the limit every workout.'

As many repetitions as possible (AMRAP)

AMRAP is a highly effective training method for developing strength, muscular endurance, and whole-body fitness. This brief overview will show you how to design and implement your own AMRAP sessions.

AMRAP is an abbreviation for the training methodology of completing *as many repetitions as possible*. Of all the training methodologies available to us – EMOM, HIIT, Tabata, etc., etc. – AMRAP is by far the simplest. However, don't let its low IQ dampen your desire to get more AMRAP in your regime. For what it lacks in sophistication it more than makes up in physical might.

So, what is it?

At its essence, AMRAP training is where we attempt to complete as many reps as physically possible in a pre-specified time period.

So, after participating in a progressive 10-minute warm-up, you would select either an individual exercise or multiples. Concluding this AMRAPing prerequisite, determine a duration, set a countdown timer, and away you go how many reps you achieve nobody knows!

Benefits of AMRAP training

Because AMRAPing is the ultimate in overload training, and because it's all about volume, it maximises muscular stimulation. This form of high intensity training, assuming that you adequately rest and replenish post session, offers a fast track to physiological adaptation which ultimately results in hypertrophy – that is, an increase in muscular density and size.

Another reason why you should consider making room in your regime for AMRAP sessions is because they send training productivity skyrocketing. Seriously, if you're one of those 'fitness enthusiasts' who thinks that a couple sets of bicep curls constitutes a workout, you'll quickly realise after one AMRAP session that you've not only been wasting your time all these years but also missing out on some quality keep fit.

In short, when AMRAPing you get a lot done in a short space of time.

AMRAP Frequently Asked Questions
How long should an AMRAP session last?
You can AMRAP for as little as one-minute or you can do a Forest Gump and keep going until you've got a toe-touching Socratic beard and a herd of mindless minions treading your every footstep.

'Ok smartarse,' you're probably thinking (if you're still with me), 'I'll rephrase my question. Is there a standard length of time trainers usually AMRAP for?'

Not that I'm aware of. However, 10-minutes seems to be a ubiquitously used temporal parameter across which trainers test their muscular endurance and mental determination. In a bid to substantiate that suggested duration, 10-minutes is the standard time used in Girevoy Sports competitions.

Can AMRAP develop fitness?

Yes, and in abundance. But then that should not come as a surprise. After all, AMRAPing is the ultimate in volume and overload training. And it's long since been understood that overloading the muscles triggers that much coveted physiological response called hypertrophy – known more colloquially as 'Gettin hench!' Anyway, if it's improved muscular endurance you seek, start AMRAPing ASAP.

But don't forget, AMRAP can work perfectly well with cardiovascular exercises. Pop on the rower, runner, or bike, set 10-minutes, and see how many metres you can cover.

Can AMRAP build strength?

Depends. Typically, strength is developed by combining maximal loads with prolonged periods of rest. Of course, if you plan to complete as many repetitions as possible of an exercise over 10-minutes, then the load must, by dint of necessity, be sub-maximal. If it isn't, you'll be drowning in metabolic waste before you get out of the first minute. In saying that though, you could still adopt the strength protocol and for 10-minutes attempt to accrue a collection of quality lifts. If you decide to do this ensure that you maintain a mind-set appropriate to that of someone who is going to execute a heavy lift: quality over quantity!

AMRAP how-to guide

Right then, roll your sleeves up and get ready to underpin the theory with a bit of practice. At this stage in this unnecessarily long explanation, you should possess a comprehensive understanding of both the benefits of and what constitutes AMRAP training. Now we're going to take a closer look at how to put an AMRAP session together. You'll be relieved to know that to do so is phenomenally simple.

First things first, select an exercise or range of exercises that you would like to pit your physicality against. The exercise(s) could be resistance or calisthenics, complex or simple, compound or isolation. If you select a resistance exercise – say the kettlebell jerk, an AMRAP exercise par excellence – you need now only concern yourself with the weight.

If you're new to AMRAP training, I suggest starting with a light weight and seeing how many reps you can bank in five or 10-minutes. Use this as a start point from which to develop and improve. I say this only because, if you acquiesce to enthusiasm, and chose too heavy a weight, you'll wind up fatiguing your muscles before getting out of the first minute.

So, to recap, when devising an AMRAP session consider the following protocol:

- Select an exercise or exercises.
- Decide on the time duration of your AMRAP – 5- or 10-minutes are best times.
- Select a weight that is commensurate with your current strength. The weight should not be too heavy nor too light, but just right so that it poses a challenge yet doesn't prohibit completion of the AMRAP.
- Participate in a thorough, whole-body warm-up that includes a cardiovascular element – such a rowing – and a series of resistance exercises (probably those that feature in your AMRAP).
- Set a countdown timer, prepare yourself mentally, and away you go . . .

EMOM training

EMOM is an abbreviation for the training methodology of completing a specific number of exercise repetitions *Every Minute On the Minute*. Though a deceptively simple form of training, it is extremely effective for a multitude of reasons.

Because it is fiercely time constrained, EMOM brings some serious military-style discipline to a training session. When you set that timer – to count either up or down – it's like having a drill sergeant in the room; and woe betide the weakling who fails to initiate the next set the moment the second's hand strikes 0:59!

Also, EMOM significantly improves training efficiency (so long as you stick to timings of course). Why? After you've completed your set number of repetitions, say 10 barbell thrusters, there is usually only just enough time on the clock to recover before the minute elapses thus triggering the next set. During an EMOM session there's no time to update your social media account or flirt with your reflection.

Furthermore, when EMOMing you can shift a shed load of weight – even over relatively short sessions. Let's say that you're time strapped and can only squeeze in a 20-minute sesh. So, you decide to complete 10 thrusters with a 40kg barbell on the minute for 20-consecutive-minutes. If you did so you'd not only bank some quality cardio, but you'd also lift a combined weight of 8,000kgs! (10 X 40kg = 400kg x 10 = 4,000kg x 2 = 8,000kg (or 8 metric ton)).

That's some going in 20-minutes.

EMOM Frequently Asked Questions
What is the purpose of EMOM?
EMOM workouts dramatically improve focus while also increasing output and exercise volume. Because they are strictly structured around the inexorable ticking of a clock, EMOM training reduces time wasted between sets.

Remembering back to your last gym session, if it was a 'conventional' workout you no doubt would have completed a number of reps, for a number of sets, for a number of exercises. That is the standard resistance training formula: reps, rest, repeat.

And while there's nothing necessarily wrong with this type of workout, the lack of time pressure can lead to exercise procrastination and with it a lot of time being wasted between sets.

When applying an EMOM framework, once you have completed the set number of reps, the remaining time is for recovery. Thus, the moment that buzzer sounds, you must get straight back into your next set. In an EMOM workout, rest periods are both limited and clearly demarcated.

What are the benefits of an EMOM workout?

There are many benefits to EMOM training. But, keeping with the ethos of EMOM, I'll sum up the benefits in a quick list.

Ten benefits of EMOM workouts

1. They are time-efficient
2. They're adaptable to most forms of training – strength, muscular endurance, cardio
3. They force you to challenge yourself
4. They can help build strength and whole-body fitness
5. They make tracking progress easy
6. They bring structure to your workouts
7. They increase training discipline
8. They improve training productivity
9. They enhance focus and motivating
10. They can even be integrated into sports

How does EMOM work?

EMOM workouts are bewilderingly easy to design. First, you need to select an exercise (or multiple exercises). The exercise could be resistance, body weight, cardiovascular, or a combination of the three. But, for ease of explanation, let's say that you decided to focus your EMOM workout on deadlifts.

Once you've made your exercise choice, you now need to settle on a weight and target rep count. This is where you must be a little bit careful. If you get carried away and select too high a weight or rep target (or both!), it's unlikely that you'll be able to complete the reps with sufficient time on the clock to recover.

It's for this reason that it is best to set a weight and rep count that can be completed in around 30-seconds. This is more important during the early stages of the EMOM workout. By setting the intensity too high too early you will unlikely make it to the final minute.

However, as you progress into the final minutes, you can reduce the rest period by increasing the reps and/or weights. This will increase the intensity thus making the workout more challenging.

After you've settled on the exercise, the weight, and rep target, all that's left is to decide how many minutes you are going for. Good EMOM workout times can range from 10-minutes up to one-hour. Though it's not set in stone, EMOM times typically increase in five-minute increments: 10-minutes, 15-minutes, 20-minutes, and so on.

Can EMOM training build muscle?
Yes, EMOM workouts can build muscle – but only if you select the right resistance exercises and appropriate weight. For example, if your EMOM workout was comprised of body weight exercises and cardio sprints, then they would not stimulate the necessary physiological adaptations that result in hypertrophy.

To encourage hypertrophy, the biological process of manufacturing more muscle tissue, you would have to focus your EMOM workouts on heavy strength exercises, such as deadlifts, bench press, squats, bent-over rows, cleans, standing shoulder press. The many EMOM workouts that feature throughout this book include a mix of muscle building and fitness developing exercises.

Circuit/workout design

There is no set component of fitness or exercise modality to which a circuit must adhere. They can, for example, be comprised entirely of cardiovascular exercises. Such a circuit would consist of various distances of running, cycling, rowing, and/or skipping. The trainer would circumnavigate the cardio loop taking little to no rest. By contrast, circuits featuring exclusively resistance exercises offer a physically demanding variation and they can also, surprisingly, induce an intense cardio workout.

When you do start to design your own circuits, there is but one basic rule to follow. And that is the rest period must always remain low. It is common among trainers to rest for as long as three-minutes between sets. Accumulatively those many rest breaks equate to a lot of missed training opportunities. Within that time a competent circuit trainer could have performed hundreds of additional reps and covered thousands of additional metres. Thus, the circuit trainer is not only utilising their time more effectively but maximising the benefits they derive from the workout. This outcome is the quintessence of circuit training.

To conclude

Limited pages and the reader's limited patience prohibit further discussion concerning the multifaceted concept of circuit design. Shame because there is so much left to be said. An entire book could be composed on the theoretical underpinnings of this underrated training method. Circuits are that versatile. But the concise encapsulations above should serve the purpose of providing you with ideas and insights into how to create your own designs. When you do put together your own circuit, be so good as to email me a copy at so that I can have a go (www.hungry4fitness.co.uk). Thanks in advance!

Appendix B
Stretching Plan

Stretching is an essential component of any exercise regime. Yet, even though it is one of the most important phases of a fitness session, few people stretch after a workout. This is a mistake. In addition to improving exercise performance, stretching is a form of self-therapy that can reduce injury susceptibility. More elastic muscles that boast a greater range of movement (ROM) are less likely to succumb to strains, pulls, and tears.

Stretching, as I see it, is like paying insurance. Something that isn't immediately pleasant but offers a measure of future protection. But the cost of this insurance cover is comparatively cheap when weighed against the potential protection it provides. A mere 10-minutes of daily stretching can confer the many benefits outlined in the following list.

Benefits of stretching
- ✓ Most importantly, regular stretching can reduce injury susceptibility.
- ✓ A consistent stretching regime can, over time, improve body alignment and posture.
- ✓ Reduces the severity of the DOMS (delayed onset of muscles soreness).
- ✓ Improves body control and awareness.
- ✓ Greater increase in range of movement (ROM) around the joint.
- ✓ Stretching improves mood.

(List adapted from: Nelson G. A, Kokkonsen, J. (2007) *Stretching Anatomy*. Human Kinetics. United States of America.)

The whole-body stretching plan below will enable you to satisfy the basic minimum recommended daily requirement of 10-minutes. Concluding every circuit and workout, set aside some time to complete the seven stretches below. Of course, you can modify, adapt, and tailor the plan to accommodate your stretching preferences. Prior to implementing the plan, familiarise yourself with the dos and don'ts of stretching so that you know how to apply safe stretching principles.

The dos and don'ts of stretching is very simple yet practical advice that if adhered to can make stretching more enjoyable and much safer. Read over the following list and incorporate the advice into your stretching routine.

The dos and don'ts of stretching

Dos	Don'ts
✓ Before applying the stretch take a deep breath and then exhale as you slowly ease into the position. ✓ Always relax into your stretch. ✓ While holding the stretch position breathe slowly as this helps ease tension. ✓ Stretch on a comfortable surface such as a soft Yoga mat. ✓ When stretching be mindful of what you are doing and concentrate on the muscle being stretched. ✓ Timing your stretches with a watch, not counting Mississippies or elephants, will ensure each stretch is applied for equal durations.	⊗ Never bounce in the stretch position. ⊗ Do not force a stretch to the point where it causes an uncomfortable pain in the muscle. ⊗ While stretching never push or put any pressure against a locked joint. ⊗ Do not rush your stretching regime. ⊗ Do not hold your breath during a stretch. ⊗ Do not allow another person to apply or assist your stretch.

The Stretches

Posterior deltoid, trapezius, and triceps

Hold the arm across the body as demonstrated in the image. The arm being stretched should remain parallel to the floor. Use your other arm to support the position.

Primary muscles stretched:
Posterior deltoid, trapezius, and trapezius

Secondary muscles stretched:
Posterior deltoid, middle and lower trapezius, rhomboids and latissimus dorsi

Apply the stretch twice on each arm for 30-seconds.

Total stretch time: 2-minutes

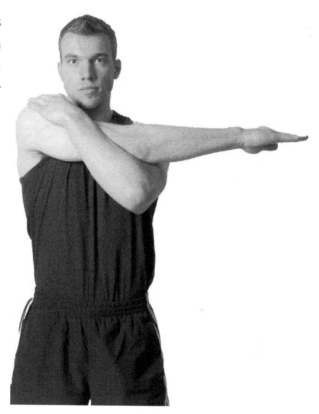

Pectoralis and biceps

Stand side on to a wall and place the hand of the arm to be stretched behind you. The arm should be pressing against the wall and parallel to the floor. Gently ease into the stretch by rotating your torso away from the wall.

Primary muscles stretched:
Pectoralis and biceps

Secondary muscles stretched:
Anterior deltoid

Apply the stretch twice on each arm for 30-seconds.

Total stretch time: 2-minutes

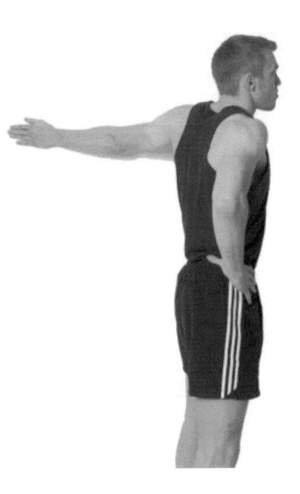

Latissimus dorsi and trapezius

Stand with feet shoulder-width apart, place the hands out in front with one clasped over the other. Keeping the arms slightly bent, push the hands away from the body rounding the back as you do so.

Primary muscles stretched: Latissimus dorsi and trapezius

Secondary muscles stretched: Rhomboids, teres major and minor

Apply the stretch twice for 30-seconds each set.

Total stretch time: 1-minute

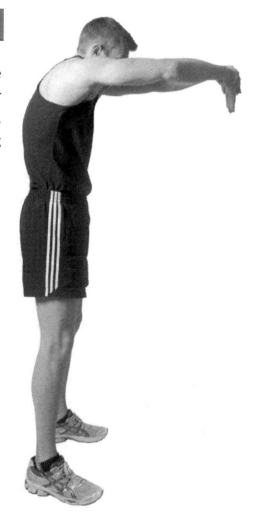

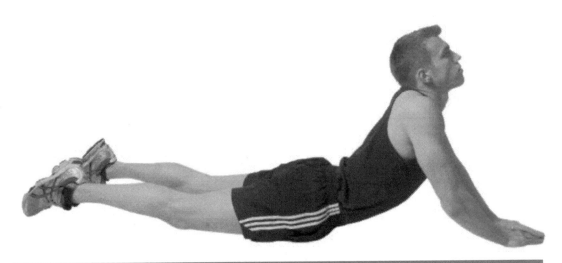

Rectus abdominals and hip flexors

Lie face down on a training mat. Place the hands and forearms on the mat either side of your face. Slowly push away from the floor until you experience a mild stretching sensation in the abdominals. When you feel the stretch in the abdominals hold the position. To increase the stretch, look up to the ceiling.

Primary muscles stretched: Rectus abdominus, external oblique, and hip flexors

Secondary muscles stretched: Internal oblique, quadratus lumborum, psoas major, iliacus, rotators and intertransversarii

Apply the stretch twice for 30-seconds per set.

Total stretch time: 1-minute

Quadriceps

Grasp onto the foot of the leg that is to be stretched. If you find it a struggle to maintain balance, use the free hand to stabilise the position. Both knees should be directly in line, slightly spaced, and the supporting leg remains bent. To apply the stretch ease the hips forwards.

Primary muscles stretched: Quadriceps

Secondary muscles stretched: Vastus intermedius, rectus femoris, psoas major, middle and upper sartorius and gluteus medius

Apply the stretch twice for 30-seconds on each leg.

Total stretch time: 2-minutes

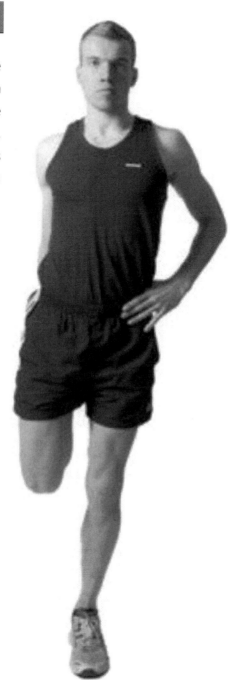

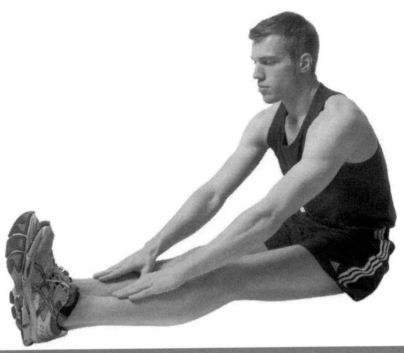

Hamstrings and gluteus maximus

Sit on a soft mat. The legs remain pressed together during the stretch and the toes point to the ceiling. Place the hands on the shins and slowly ease forward until you feel a mild stretch sensation in the back of the legs. Avoid rounding the spine and do not apply excessive force. This is a severe stretching position and thus should be performed carefully.

Primary muscles stretched: Hamstrings and gluteus maximus

Secondary muscles stretched: Semitendinosus, semimembranosus, biceps femoris, gastrocnemius, lower erector spinae

Apply the stretch twice for 30-seconds each set.

Total stretch time: 1-minute

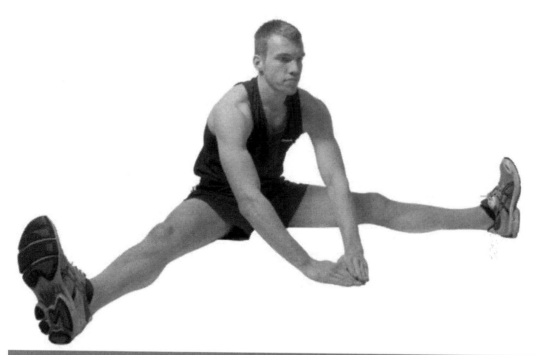

Hamstrings and adductors

Again, sit on a soft mat. Spread the legs open until you can feel a mild stretch creep into the hamstrings. The toes should be pointing up towards the ceiling and the back must remain straight throughout. Place the hands on the floor and slowly rotate the pelvis forward. To amplify the intensity of the stretch you can also lean forward.

Primary muscles stretched: Hamstrings and adductors

Secondary muscles stretched: Semitendinosus, semimembranosus, gracilis, adductor magnus and longus, gluteus maximus, lower erector spinae, lower latissimus dorsi, medial side of soleus, medial and lateral head of gastrocnemius

Apply this stretch twice for 30-seconds each set.

Total stretch time: 1-minute

References

Bean, A. (2008). *Strength Training: The Complete Guide To.* A & C Black. London.

Greger, M. Stone, G. (2017). *How Not to Die*. USA. Macmillan.

Little, J. (1998). *The Art of Expressing The Human Body*. Tuttle Publishing. USA.

McArdle, W. D., Katch, F. I., Katch, V. L. (2001). *Exercise Physiology Fifth Edition*. Lippincott, Williams & Wilkins.

Nelson, G. A, Kokkonsen, J. (2007). *Stretching Anatomy.* Human Kinetics. United States of America.

Schwarzenegger, A. (1998). *The Encyclopaedia Of Modern Bodybuilding.* Simon & Schuster. New York.

Shepherd, J. (2006). *Sports Training: The Complete Guide To*. A&C Black. London.

Tsatsouline, P. (2001). *The Russian Kettlebell Challenge*. Dragon Door Publications. USA.

Watson, A. W. S. (1995). *Physical Fitness & Athletic Performance*. Longman. England.

Made in the USA
Las Vegas, NV
07 July 2023

74319485R00162